Feminist Therapy Theory and Practice

Mary Ballou, PhD, ABPP, is a professor of counseling psychology at Northeastern University, the chair of the Feminist Therapy Institute, an ABPP diplomate in counseling psychology, and an APA fellow. She is the counseling psychology program director at Northeastern University and practices counseling and consultation in Boston and in Keene, New Hampshire. She has published many books and articles and has contributed chapters to many texts. Mary is a many-generation Yankee who has helped raise two girls while practicing, teaching, writing, and working toward change in several professional and local organizations. She experiences her identities most clearly when endeavoring to live life congruently with her principles.

Marcia Hill, EdD, is a woman of primarily northern European ancestry in her late 50s. Her parents were professionals, and although they valued education, resources were limited, and she was expected to fund her own education. She did so by working, choosing inexpensive schools, and procuring loans and scholarships. She found her way into psychology "sideways." In her life experiences, women worked as homemakers, clerical workers, nurses, or teachers. Because she was an ambitious child, that left teaching or nursing, and her mother, a nurse, warned her away from nursing. Marcia's career path went from special education to English education to school psychology and finally to clinical psychology. When she first arrived at school, she had barely heard of therapy and certainly did not know anyone who had been to a therapist. She came into feminism as the second wave was first starting, in about 1969, and felt as though the world finally made sense. Her feminism has thus been part of her vision and practice of therapy from the outset.

She is in private practice in Vermont. She has edited ten books about various aspects of feminist therapy and is the author of *Diary of a Country Therapist* (1994).

Carolyn West, PhD, writes from the perspective of a 61-year-old Caucasian woman of western European heritage. She was raised during the 1950s in small town in New England and internalized messages from her family and community and the larger culture regarding the place of children and women and the status of the nonprofessional class. During this time and in this place, being seen (only in proscribed ways) but not heard was an expectation not only for children. Carolyn is also a single mother, and this latter status is largely responsible for the tipping point of oppressive discomfort that propelled her toward a standpoint from which she could name the factors affecting her development and choices and from which she now attempts to assist others in this regard.

Feminist Therapy Theory and Practice

A Contemporary Perspective

Mary Ballou, PhD, ABPP,
Marcia Hill, EdD, and
Carolyn West, PhD

Editors

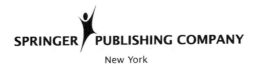

SPRINGER PUBLISHING COMPANY

New York

Springer Publishing Company, LLC
11 West 42nd Street
New York, NY 10036
www.springerpub.com

Acquisitions Editor: Sheri W. Sussman
Production Editor: Megan Timian
Cover design: Joanne E. Honigman
Composition: Publication Services

07 08 09 10/5 4 3 2 1

Library of Congress Cataloging-in-Publication Data

Feminist therapy theory and practice : a contemporary perspective / Mary Ballou, Marcia Hill,
Carolyn West, editors.
    p. ; cm.
  Includes bibliographical references and index.
  ISBN 978-0-8261-1957-5 (hardcover : alk. paper)
  1. Feminist therapy. I. Ballou, Mary B., 1949- II. Hill, Marcia. III. West, Carolyn M. (Carolyn
Marie)
  [DNLM: 1. Feminism. 2. Psychotherapy. 3. Models, Psychological. 4. Psychological Theory.
5. Women's Health. WM 420 F3295 2008]

RC489.F45F48 2008
616.89'14—dc22
                                      2007041553

Printed in the United States of America by Edwards Brothers, Inc.

This book is dedicated to the continuity of collaboration
in the development of feminist therapy, past, present, and future,
with a special acknowledgment to Jean Baker Miller.

Table of Contents

Contributors

Susan Barrett, PhD, has been in independent practice as a psychotherapist in Atlanta, Georgia, since 1980. Prior to that, in 1974, she cofounded and worked at Karuna: Counseling for Women and Their Friends, a feminist therapy center. She has been a member of the Feminist Therapy Institute since its inception in 1982. She sees herself as an applied theorist, weaving back and forth between theoretical frameworks and the lived experience of people, including focusing her doctoral work on understanding psychological empowerment as a theoretical framework for feminist therapy. She was raised as the oldest of six children in a white, middle-class, educated, stable Catholic family. After coming through the women's movement and coming out as a lesbian in the early 1970s, she is now firmly embedded in her bicultural and biracial immediate family of a partner and two children and her broader network of extended family and friends. Living in her adopted South, she struggles to keep one foot in psychology and one in social change efforts.

Lauren Gentile, MS, is a third-year doctoral student at Northeastern University. She currently works as a practicum student at Fenway Community Health Center, where she sees members of the Fenway gay, lesbian, bisexual, and transgender (GLBT) community for individual counseling. She also facilitates a 15-week coming-out support group. Lauren hopes to continue to use a feminist framework in her writing and clinical practice.

Mary Margaret Hart, PhD, is a woman in her mid-50s, of white European descent. She grew up Catholic in New Jersey, the oldest child of Midwestern parents who were never fully at home on the East Coast. Education was strongly valued in her family, and she graduated from Trenton State College and then received a master's degree in psychology from Duquesne University. She received her PhD from Penn State University in 1980 and taught human development at Penn State until 1986, when she entered full-time practice as a psychotherapist (psychologist), beginning in a community mental health setting and moving on to her current private practice in rural central Pennsylvania.

She first identified herself as a feminist in the early 1970s, had two daughters in the mid-1970s, and identified as lesbian in the late 1970s. Her experiences of herself as a woman, a mother, and a lesbian have formed the core of her personal identity. Her personal understanding of the often oppressive nature of social structures and institutionalized power was most profoundly formed in the context of the fear she experienced for years of losing her children because of her identification with a group defined by the dominant culture as abnormal and inferior.

Jae Y. Jeong, MS, has been, for as long as she can remember, aware of the power of race, socioeconomic status, fluency in the English language, and adversity. Born in South Korea, she immigrated with her family to the United States in 1983. Obtaining a well-rounded education and developing artistic talents were emphasized in this educated immigrant family. Her journey toward psychology was guided by observations of recovery and personal transformations that were left unexplained by medicine alone. In her master's program, she developed a relationship with her mentor, which she cites as one of the most influential experiences in her personal life and professional career. She was challenged to reconsider traditional approaches to well-being and to incorporate an ecological systems framework that integrates issues of diversity and multiculturalism with feminist perspectives and value systems.

Susie Kisber, PysD, is a clinical psychologist living in the San Francisco Bay area with her partner. Their family of choice includes children they did not bear who are growing up exposed to many examples of gender fluidity. She describes herself as a white, Jewish, bisexual woman who was raised upper middle class in Atlanta and was born during the civil rights movement. As a result of becoming disabled at the age of 3 and being a fourth-generation Southern Jew, she experienced difference and marginalization while also having access to class power and privilege. From an early age, she became interested in people's experience of difference and in how power and privilege play out.

Elaine Leeder, PhD, is the dean of social sciences at Sonoma State University in Rohnert Park, California. She was trained as a social worker and has a master's in public health and a PhD in sociology. Her newest book, *Inside and Out: Women, Prison and Therapy,* was published in 2007. Her other books include *Rose Pesotta: Anarchist and Labor Organizer* (1993), *Treating Abuse in Families: A Feminist and Community Approach* (Springer, 1994), and *The Family in Global Perspective: A Gendered Journey* (2003). Leeder is the daughter of a Holocaust survivor, which has informed all of her work fighting social inequities, and is the mother of an activist, feminist, and drama therapist. The work goes on into the next generation.

Liz Margolies, MSW, is a social worker living and practicing in New York City. Coming of age in the 1970s, her work has always been grounded in a social justice perspective. In addition to her private practice, she coordinates a volunteer mediation service, directs a bereavement program at three animal hospitals, teaches social justice at Fordham University Graduate School of Social Service, and serves as the therapeutic consultant for the Donor Sibling Registry. She is also the founder and executive director of the LGBT Cancer Project, the country's first program devoted exclusively to the needs of LGBT people with cancer and those at risk. She has written essays, training manuals, and numerous scholarly articles on women and mental health. Woven around all these work projects, Liz is a devoted single parent of a 15-year-old son named Wolfe. She is, as a social worker, devoted to and trained in the work of social justice.

Mary Ni, EdD, is a 57-year-old, first-generation Chinese American. She grew up trying to assimilate "white." After college, books such as *Women and Madness* (Phyllis Chesler), *Towards a New Psychology of Women* (Jean Baker Miller), *The Second Sex* (Simone de Beauvoir), and *The Divided Self* (R. D. Laing) informed her thinking and raised her feminist consciousness in ways that her formal education had not. Through reevaluation co-counseling (RC) activities—a type of ongoing non-therapy, yet therapeutic, peer-helping arrangement (Harvey Jackins)—she experienced the powerful and transformative results that can occur from sharing uncensored personal stories in a safe community. In that context, she developed a heightened understanding of socially oppressive systems and the possibilities for organized personal and social change. She also realized the healing possibilities in peer groups for people who would not seek (or might not be able to afford) private therapy. Her contribution to this book is influenced by this perspective.

Claudia Pitts, PhD, is a clinical psychologist who balances life as both a clinician and an academic. She works at a private practice in suburban Chicago and is on the psychology faculty at National-Louis University. Her training is "traditional," and her understanding as a feminist therapist has evolved since graduate school. She views her work as faculty, at a university with an exceptionally diverse student body, as a way to promote social justice. She also strives to reflect these values in her clinical work.

Eleanor Roffman, EdD, is a professor at Lesley University in the counseling and psychology division of the Graduate School of Arts and Social Sciences.

As a feminist activist for over 30 years, she has worked in the areas of violence toward women, access to equal education, housing concerns, and the role of psychology in addressing the needs of women, children, and people in poor communities. She frequently consults internationally, most recently using the expressive arts to address trauma in both Palestine and Cambodia. A particular focus for her has been the international solidarity movement for peace and justice in the Middle East. Her publications address feminist pedagogy, clinical supervision, international women's issues, and a feminist perspective on social class. Feminism grounds her clinical, academic, and activist achievements.

Jaime Suvak, MS, a licensed mental health counselor, currently works at the Boston Area Rape Crisis Center (BARCC) as the clinical training manager. She has been working to end sexual violence and support survivors for over 10 years. She began at the Centre County Resource Center in Pennsylvania as a volunteer. In the past 5 years, she has directed both the hotline and the medical advocacy programs at BARCC. She is currently developing and presenting trainings for professionals throughout Boston communities. Suvak has been a member of FTI since 2002 and hopes to continue to work within the framework of feminist therapy as well as share the importance of it with others.

Charity Tabol, MS, is a doctoral candidate in the Department of Counseling and Applied Educational Psychology at Northeastern University and is a new steering committee member of the Feminist Therapy Institute. Charity has worked clinically with a wide variety of individuals in hospital, outpatient, and forensic settings, and she currently works at a Veterans Affairs (VA) hospital in Bedford, Massachusetts. She strives to adhere to feminist principles and ethics in her therapeutic encounters and other aspects of her work, even while immersed in traditional medical-model settings. She also works for social change in her "outside" life through writing and volunteerism. She has a burgeoning interest in the effects of power disparities and other coercive influences on trainees and beginning therapists and psychologists who are attempting to find their own voice.

Gail Walker, PhD, ADTR, LPC, is in private practice in Kendall Park, New Jersey. Using her training in psychological counseling and movement/dance therapy, she explores the interface of mind, emotion, body, spirit, and community with her clients. She offers training in internalized oppression, relational/cultural theory, sexuality, and therapy issues specific to chronic and life-threatening illness. For 30 years she has walked the dual paths of feminism and spirituality and has built bridges between them.

Several additional members of the Feminist Therapy Institute also contributed to the development of this book through their participation in discussions at the Advanced Therapy Institute (AFTI) meeting in Dayton, Ohio, in 2007. Women who contributed to the development of the text through the AFTI discussion included Juli Burnell, Marnie Leavitt, Tina Kaljevic, and Brithany Kawloski.

Gail Anderson, Liz Margolies, and Denny Webster wrote the cases discussed throughout the application chapters.

Preface

THE CONTEXT OF THIS VOLUME

The original *Handbook of Feminist Therapy* was published over 20 years ago, in 1985. Feminist therapy was in its youth, perhaps 15 years old at best. Social workers had long politicized poverty, but it was new to politicize gender and to incorporate that perspective into the practice of psychotherapy. The handbook was a somewhat random collection of articles, with each topic a contribution to the literature, so sparse was any writing in the area. The focus was almost exclusively on gender, with some attention to sexual orientation. Much has changed.

In the more than 20 years intervening, feminist therapy has evolved its understanding of oppression to include attention to race and ethnicity, class, disability, age, and the many other dimensions of politicized difference. Gender and sexual orientation are no longer assumed to be binary. From a primary focus on the misuse of sex as a weapon, the theory and practice of feminist therapy has become more sex-positive in general. Feminist therapy principles have been applied to diverse populations, from women in prison (Harden & Hill, 1998; Leeder, 2006) to women in the former Yugoslavia (Sharratt & Kaschak, 1999) to children (Anderson & Hill, 1997) and many others. Authors and researchers have looked at money (Hill & Kaschak, 1999), ethics (Kaschak & Hill, 1999; Rave & Larsen, 1995), class (Hill & Rothblum, 1996), disability (Olkin, 2005), and numerous other topics through the lens of feminist therapy.

Additionally, much of feminist thinking has been incorporated into mainstream psychotherapy training and ethics and even into legislation. Domestic violence, childhood sexual abuse, rape, and sexual harassment are more frequently recognized and reported; police and hospitals are trained to respond; and resources exist to assist those who have experienced these crimes. Professional codes of ethics encourage cultural competence and are clearer about boundary violations. Articles with a feminist perspective, once ghettoized into feminist publications, now appear regularly in mainstream professional journals. In what is perhaps both a compliment and an insult, ideas taken from feminist therapy (but without acknowledgment) have found their way into much of the literature on therapy.

In this context, and with an additional 20-plus years of work, feminist therapy has become increasingly sophisticated, and the conceptualization of this book reflects that. Rather than a collection of articles on a variety of topics, this volume is organized in a way that brings the reader through an overview of thinking in feminist therapy. The text is divided into five sections.

THE ORGANIZATION OF THIS VOLUME

We begin by looking at the context of therapy. Therapy in the United States is embedded in the particular culture of this country in this period of time. Who is therapy for, especially in this age of managed care and focus on corporate profits? What we look at (and don't look at) in therapy, how we arrange payment, and how we diagnose the problem all are part of the context of therapy. In addition, feminists now have allies: other schools of thought or social movements with which we stand in at least some mutual solidarity. These also are part of feminist therapy's context today.

Next, we consider the person who comes to therapy. How do we look at who this person is in the context of her or his many identities? We consider the tension between recognizing the specific concerns and struggles of particular groups and honoring the specificity of the individual.

Then we examine psychotherapy itself with a feminist lens. The feminist therapist works at many levels simultaneously—the individual, the relational and community, and the sociostructural—and shifts focus freely among them. Feminism has informed a variety of approaches and techniques, and this will also be discussed.

Ethics and activism are central to a feminist perspective, and this is part of what sets feminist therapy apart from other approaches. A therapy theory that is grounded in an understanding of political harm as part of what brings people to therapy cannot be understood separately from political action.

Finally, we put all the pieces—the context, the client, practice, and activism—together and consider what the integration of these elements would entail. Given all of these pieces, how do we think about what causes human suffering and what we as therapists can do about it?

Each of these sections consists of two paired chapters, one looking at theory and the second describing application of that theory. Thus, we move from concept to practice in each section. In addition, we have developed three case examples, so that the practice chapters can give a human face to their discussion of what feminist therapy practice would actually look like. You will follow the cases of Anna and Sergei, Abby, and Scott through the book's application chapters.

Feminist therapy is remarkably richer, more complex and nuanced, than it was 20 years ago. We welcome you as you consider what it has to offer.

REFERENCES

Anderson, G., & Hill, M. (Eds.). (1997). Children's rights, therapists' responsibilities. *Women and Therapy, 20*(2).

Harden, J., & Hill, M. (Eds.). (1998). Breaking the rules: Women in prison and feminist therapy. *Women and Therapy, 20*(4), *21*(1).

Hill, M., & Kaschak, E. (Eds.). (1999). For love or money: The fee in feminist therapy. *Women and Therapy, 22*(3).

Hill, M., & Rothblum, E. (Eds.). (1996). Classism and feminist therapy: Counting the costs. *Women and Therapy, 18*(3–4).

Kaschak, E., & Hill, M. (Eds.). (1999). Beyond the rule book: Moral issues and dilemmas in the practice of psychotherapy. *Women and Therapy, 22*(2).

Leeder, E. (Ed.). (2006). Inside and out: Women, prison and therapy. *Women and Therapy, 29*(3–4).

Olkin, R. (2005). Women with disabilities. In J. C. Chrisler, C. Golden, & P. D. Rosee (Eds.), *Lectures on the psychology of women* (3rd ed.). New York: McGraw-Hill.

Rave, E., & Larsen, E. (1995). *Ethical decision making in therapy feminist perspectives.* New York: Guilford Press.

Sharratt, S., & Kaschak, E. (Eds.). (1999). Assault on the soul: Women in the former Yugoslavia. *Women and Therapy, 22*(1).

Introduction: From There to Here

FEMINIST THERAPY'S BEGINNINGS

Feminist therapy was first named and developed in the late 1970s and early 1980s as the second wave of feminism penetrated the awareness of professionals and academics. It had already touched so-inclined students and activists. Other challenging forces and influences of that era were also part of the storm, such as the civil rights and gay rights movements; antiwar efforts, including Students for a Democratic Society; the use of drugs in pursuit of recreation and insight; and the human potential movement. Liberation movements had substantial impact, and the awareness generated then continues today. All of these factors served as notice that social values in the United States were entering a progressive era.

Mental health theory and practice then were not so strongly coupled with the medical model and with empirical science. Indeed, practice was informed largely by psychodynamic theory, with pockets of humanism. While theoretical physics was grappling with relativity and systems theory, and the first interdisciplinary women's studies programs were exciting many in academia, behaviorism was the innovative theory building on the underpinning of logical positivist research in academic psychology. In departments of psychology, clinical psychology was an uncomfortable graduate specialty with clear preference for psychometrics and demands for solid preparation in the science of human behavior. In psychiatry the *Diagnostic and Statistical Manual, Third Edition (DSM-III)*, with its specified criteria for mental health problems, was being developed with claims of improving the validity and reliability of the diagnoses of mental illness. However, it did not yet rule thinking (and payment) in therapy and counseling. Schools of social work varied; some supported current social policy while seeking to develop clinical psychiatric programs, whereas schools with more progressive politics (e.g., Brandeis University and the University of Michigan) formulated social theory and engaged in penetrating and wide-ranging policy critiques. Counselor education programs flourished, having been funded in the 1950s through National Defense Act grants for the purpose of guiding school children to study science and math so they could contribute to the Cold War effort. These guidance programs matured into counselor education training programs that were solidly based in humanistic and developmental orientations.

Yet in this same era, people stimulated by the cross-fertilization of developing theory and grassroots practices were discussing the art and science of therapy, the impact of social psychology and women's psychology, and community-based responses to the crises and needs of the times. The anti-psychiatry and radical psychiatry movements challenged conventional views by raising political issues about status and the social and economic aspects of racial discrimination. Volunteers trained in helping skills, worked in grassroots programs for victims of rape and domestic violence, or staffed suicide and drug hotlines. These centers operated largely outside of local government or professional mental health services. In fact most crisis support programs were outside of formal physical and mental health systems. Although relationships between volunteer services and hospital emergency rooms were quick to develop in this era, the two were autonomous.

Feminist therapy developed in this fertile milieu. Feminist therapy's insistence on analyzing power and gender roles, on attending to and sharing power in counseling, and on always taking into account the damage done to women by a sexist society drew from and contributed to other forces of the times. It was an exciting and open time, when community groups and some academics were engaged in newer and germinal thinking and innovative development.

THE INFLUENCE OF TODAY'S POLITICAL CLIMATE

Feminist therapy continues to be used today, yet in a very different context. Thirty years have brought many developments in paradigms; in academic, professional, and social ideologies; and in economic systems and ruling structures. Today's values and social policies have become sharply more conservative. Although some movement into a postindustrial capitalism has occurred, it is not yet clear who will benefit and who will be harmed in the global economic shift to advanced capitalism. Both technology and the drive for new markets have had a dramatic impact on international politics and the shifting grounds on which the old structures of social order sit. For example, immigration policies in the United States, always influenced by economic and political factors, are now overtly shaped, at least in the media, by exclusionary perspectives. The "culture wars" give evidence that conservative ideology has strengthened and gained force in setting the social policy and political agenda, and economic status is a much more obvious influence in the motivations of our times.

This conservative turn is also felt in the mental health professions, in universities, and in human services. Funding for social services has been systematically cut, and private services have been encouraged. For example, the recent change in welfare policy will allow dramatic cuts to social service budgets, even while funds for the military increase. This has served to effectively shift the resources from human need to corporate profit. The "No Child Left Behind" educational policies are another example. Although it is noble to be concerned with the learning of each child in our society, when learning is defined, measured, and funded—to the degree that it *is* funded—solely on the basis of performance on standardized achievement tests, this is a very narrow understanding of learning. And most telling is the underside of this current social policy—castaway students who do not perform in ways deemed acceptable by those privileged to set the standards. The professions have contributed to these exclusionary practices, as can be seen in several recent developments. Creating disorders and specialists to treat the problems is seen in early childhood interventions. As economic support for mental health service is reduced, and private hospitals and practices become controlled by private profit corporations, clinical psychologists are looking for positions in the schools. Universities are becoming increasingly driven by money. Tuition costs are increasing, as are demands on faculty to do research that is externally funded; and approval of programs is based in large part on whether they will generate enough dollars to make a profit.

Professionals too are affected by these trends. Most of the major professional organizations, now far from the original concept of being learned societies, currently need to act as political action committees (PACs) and network with the government at national and state levels. They seek inclusion of their profession—and too often the exclusion of others—in licensing laws, in standards of best practices, and as named professions in funding legislation.

Theory building and research have become much more narrowly focused. Mainstream theories in psychology and psychiatry have ignored or trivialized important social, economic, and structural influences on people and retreated to theories that once again focus on individual development of disorders brought about through biological, neurological, and genetic factors, or problems with thoughts and behaviors. Thus, some version of problems in behavior or biology underlies most of the dominant theory. This sort of reduction is very much in keeping with the domination of logical positivist research, which presumes that material reality can be clearly and consistently measured by instruments that compare well to already existing instruments. The goal is to generate group averages so that individuals then can be compared to a standard. This is a powerful method, and in its place, among other methods of inquiry, it can be valuable. However, much in mental health is not material, and individuals do and should differ. Further, there is much that influences people that is not based in biology or faulty thinking and is thus excluded from consideration. Our theories and the ways of inquiry are very narrow in mental health in this era.

THE CRISIS IN HEALTH CARE

Health care in general and mental health care in particular have serious problems in the United States today. Many consider it a crisis. Health insurance is usually tied to employment, and it costs too much for individuals and employers. Many employees cannot afford escalating insurance, and employers either provide none or require employees to pay increasingly large portions of the insurance cost. Little effort is currently being exerted to contain sharply rising health care costs.

Many people go without any insurance at all. Receiving no services or relying on emergency services has become increasingly common. The effectiveness of emergency services is impaired by such demand. These deficiencies force attention to acute illness after it has already passed preventable stages. For example, people often try to numb fear and hopelessness with legal prescriptions, or illegal drugs. If our mental health system were more effective, preventive counseling and social supports would be authorized and available. But instead, more typically we see ill people in prisons or rotating in and out of acute units for drug stabilization. Another dimension of the crisis in health care is the nearly exclusive use of a model that focuses on the individual as the site of illness. Preventive approaches and recognition of the structural and environmental causes of individuals' ills do not fit with current U.S. health care practices. Counseling for more effective decision making, for minimizing the impact of harmful events, and for seeking support for life transitions or further growth is no longer available in the mental health system. Should such preventive and growth facilitation occur, it is self-pay and provided by counselors trained in an earlier era. Today's insurance requires criteria of medical necessity for authorization of services. Wellness, prevention, and support for life transitions are not deemed medically necessary. Access to and restriction of services are but part of the problem.

That insurance companies—for-profit corporations—should be able to control cost and services is very strange indeed. One might say "only in America"! The United States is the only major developed nation that allows health care to be controlled by for-profit corporations and through business models for corporate profit. Other countries provide quality health care as a responsibility of the government through federal and municipal services, like clean water, safe roads, and police and fire services.

Health care is big business, and it has influenced government to allow it to continue to profit despite the crisis. Attempts by professional groups, states, and advocacy groups to challenge the corporate control have been thwarted. The military, the poor, the elderly, and the disabled can already receive health care provided by or paid for through government programs. Yet the resistance to providing quality health care for all is very strong.

Today health and social services are too limited. Funds for these services have been cut, and cut again. The increase in the number of people with mental illness and the number of mentally ill people in prisons and the homeless populations is only one indication. Social service supports available at one time through federal funding have been turned over to the states with sharply reduced funding. Many social services are virtually gone, leaving few supports for those harmed by the structural problems and precipitating even more mental health problems.

Universal health care that includes supportive, growth-oriented, and preventive mental health is badly needed. Support for community-based services that can provide some of this care and for forms of care beyond individual treatment is also necessary. The answer to the crisis is clear; the direction lies ahead. Yet hegemony of the professions seeking inclusion, corporate interests, and government regulation has blocked critical movement forward.

It is a difficult time for feminist therapy. Graduate schools frequently do not have courses in or even substantial coverage of feminist therapy. New theory texts trivialize it. Empirically validated treatments exclude it. Conceptualizations of mental illness ignore external forces. Nonetheless, this is also a very important time for feminist therapy. Feminist therapy has led the way for thinking and doing therapy differently. Many other models of therapy have followed its lead in understanding the effects of sociocultural context on human suffering. The thinking and practice of feminist therapy continues, but the context of early 21st century politics in the United States makes its practice and development far more difficult.

THIRD-WAVE FEMINISM

In the 1990s and into the next decade, a new focus for feminism has emerged. This focus, the "third wave" of feminism, is just being clearly defined at present. Various groups have called for attention to their experiences as central to feminism. They claim feminist inclusion too!

Judith Lorber, in the third edition of her *Gender Inequality: Feminist Theories and Politics*, organizes her text into sections titled "Gender Reform Feminisms," "Gender Resistance Feminisms," and "Gender Rebellion Feminisms." Under these headings she includes multicultural/multiracial feminism, feminist studies of men, social construction feminism, postmodern feminism, and third-wave feminism. She states,

> The future strength of the feminist movement lies in the variety and density of multiple identities—not just Woman. The primary identity of feminists may be gender, racial ethnical group, religion, social class, or sexual orientation in some combination. The focus of feminist work may be peace, sexual violence, political parity, economic opportunity, or one of many proliferating causes. The beneficiaries may be one specific oppressed group or many. Feminist identity may be way down the list, implicit, or even masked, but as long as the perspective is critical and the goal is political, economic, and cultural equality for all, then it is feminism. (p. 322)

Wendy Kolmar and Frances Bartkowski, in their *Feminist Theory: A Reader*, provide us with several essays presenting and arguing for inclusion into contemporary feminism. Included are essays on intersectional and identity politics; cultures and postcolonial perspectives; transgender and queer theory as added to the debates on sex, sexuality, and gender; global realities—economy, migration, world trade, environmental denigration, and the militarization of women's lives; integrating disability; and the impact of medical and technological mechanization.

In the second edition of her *Feminist Theories and Feminist Psychotherapies: Origins, Themes, and Diversity*, Carolyn Zerbe Enns presents third-wave feminism a bit differently. She describes the recent developments in feminist theory as deriving from postmodernism, seeing it as coming from academic disciplines rather than from the social activism of earlier feminisms. She sees postmodernism as contributing a method for questioning the limits and embedded assumptions of knowledge, coupling this with difference and diversity. Carolyn uses lesbian and queer theory as an example of applying postmodern thinking to second-wave feminist topics. She defines the third wave of feminism as the daughter of second-wave feminists.

As the descriptions of these three notable works indicate, feminism's third wave is variously understood. What is common among these descriptions is a fresh look at issues in global and widely divergent ways. Feminism has not been stagnant. Despite the comfort of categorization, it is very clear that critical thinking and the demand for parity continues. Feminist thinkers unearthing and articulating the sociostructural factors in politics, in economics, in environmentalism, in cultural traditions, and in thinking are very present, alive, and important. It is equally clear that multiplicity and complexity are a counterpoint to controlling interests. And it is absolutely clear that power and its many abuses still are to be named and combated!

THE CASE STUDIES

This book is organized into paired theory and application chapters, with the application chapters focusing on three specific case studies. The case studies were created to offer the reader some variety in clients, contexts, and difficulties, in the hope that this would provide a small window into the great range of approaches feminist therapy embraces. In the following pages you will find these case descriptions. If you are a professional, we encourage you to imagine these people in your office: How might you assist them? If you are not a therapist, think of these people as your neighbors or friends or coworkers: what do you think they need to live more fully and comfortably?

Scott

Scott is a 9-year-old white male in the third grade whose parents are concerned about his difficulty making friends, especially with males. This blue-eyed boy is tall for his age, is about 20 pounds overweight or "chubby," has curly blond hair, and describes himself as clumsy. He states frankly that he doesn't like boys, but prefers girls as friends. When asked why, he says that boys tease him, call him "girlie-girl," and pick on him. Also, he adds that "boys do bad things to girls." There are times when Scott further alienates the boys in his class by "accidentally" tripping them when they walk by his desk or by otherwise seeking revenge behaviorally. A complaint from the school about this behavior prompted Scott's referral to therapy.

Scott likes to dress up like girls do sometimes at home and has fun with his older sister, his only sibling, playing traditional "girls' games" such as house or dolls. Scott's parents are tolerant of who he is but also have tried to help him overcome his dislike of males and have talked to him about being a "gentle male" or gentleman. Scott is a loving child most of the time and is very affectionate with family members. He is musical and enjoys playing the piano. Scott is a B student at school. He pitches in at home with chores. He comes from a religious family and goes to a church-based elementary school in a small Midwestern town. His parents are high school graduates in supervisory jobs, his mother as a restaurant manager and his father as a foreman.

His mother takes a primary role in child care, but Scott's father is also very involved and is a "gentle" man. They work opposite shifts so that a parent is usually home with the children in this emotionally close family. Extended family is not in the geographical area.

Abby

Abby is an African American woman who grew up in a small town an hour outside of the city where she now lives. Her parents divorced when she was 7. When her mother remarried 2 years later, Abby, her two brothers, and her mother moved into her stepfather's house. Life there was stable, and Abby became close with her stepfather. They shared a love of sports and often went together to watch basketball or football games in the city. One night, during the hour-long drive home from the game, Abby fell asleep in the front seat. She awoke to find her stepfather fondling her while he drove. She was shocked, confused, and ashamed. Abby pretended to remain asleep and rolled toward the window, away from her stepfather and out of his reach. They never discussed what happened. Abby remembers two other incidents of waking to find her stepfather sitting on her bed, his hand in her pajamas. Each time, she rolled away and pretended to remain asleep.

At college, Abby began drinking with friends and found that she liked the way it made her feel. She was drinking heavily by her sophomore year but reassured herself with her high grades and a promise that she would quit when she graduated. Abby successfully gave up alcohol, but her anxiety level increased with sobriety and her first job. Her primary care physician prescribed Xanax. Abby has not been without a benzodiazepine prescription since then, although her usage has fluctuated over time.

Abby began therapy after a period of recurring worry that she had left her condo door unlocked. She called for the first appointment after an incident where she had to return home at lunch to check the door. During the consultation, she also mentioned that, although she dated occasionally, she had not been in a relationship for many years. She realized that she was running out of time to have children, something she always imagined she would do. When asked about her family, Abby reported that her stepfather had recently been diagnosed with colon cancer, and she was worried about how upset her mother was.

Anna and Sergei

Anna and Sergei have been in the United States since 2000, when they left their home in Russia to start a new life. In Russia, Sergei had a job as an apprentice carpenter, and Anna worked part-time in a bakery and coffee shop. They intended to become permanent citizens of the United States, but the past few years have been so difficult for them they have been unable to pursue that goal.

They now have two small children, ages 1 and 3. The younger child, Sasha, was born with a serious cardiac condition that has necessitated several surgeries, and more are anticipated. While he was working as a carpenter this past year, Sergei was injured and had to miss so much work that he lost his job, which was the only source of health benefits for the family. Anna had been staying home with the children, but now is trying to provide income for the family by working nights cleaning offices and several days a week helping at a neighborhood bakery, while Sergei watches the children. On days when Sergei can get work indoors, a neighbor baby-sits. Both parents are worried that if they cannot pay the rent for their one-bedroom apartment, they soon will be without housing.

Anna and Sergei are devoted to each other and their children, and they continue to believe that they could succeed in the United States if they could find work that would support the family. They have made few friends in their neighborhood and have not attended a church since the children were born. There are few people in their city who speak their language or understand their circumstances. They are now worried that unless Sergei can maintain regular employment, they will be forced to return to Russia, where they would have some family support and the possibility of obtaining health care for their son. Sometimes they argue about the decision, and once, when their voices became very loud, and the children began to cry, a neighbor contacted social services to be sure the children were not being injured. This incident is what brought them to therapy.

REFERENCES

Enns, C. Z. (2004). *Feminist theories and feminist psychotherapies: Origins, themes, and diversity* (2nd ed.). New York: Haworth Press.

Kolmar, W., & Bartkowski, F. (2004). *Feminist theory: A reader* (2nd ed.). Boston: McGraw-Hill.

Lorber, J. (2005). *Gender inequality: Feminist theories and politics* (3rd ed.). Los Angeles: Roxbury.

Feminist Therapy Theory and Practice

CHAPTER 1

The Context of Therapy: *Theory*

Mary Ballou and Marcia Hill

Despite, or possibly because of, the crisis in mental health care, important feminist therapy inquiry continues. Feminism and therapy have been companions since, perhaps, Mander and Rush wrote *Feminism as Therapy* in 1974, followed by Jean Baker Miller's *Toward a New Psychology of Women*, in 1976. The liberation movements of the 1960s, the second wave of feminism (particularly in the United States), the publication in 1972 of Phyllis Chesler's exposé *Women and Madness*, grassroots consciousness-raising groups, and collectively written position papers all laid the groundwork for the emergence of feminist therapy. Rapid publication of articles and books on feminist therapy followed. Feminist therapy has been developing for over 30 years in the professional literature, and longer in women's communities. The literature is rich and varied, reflecting the vitality of feminist therapy.

FEMINIST THERAPY'S INFLUENCE ON THE FIELD

"Developing" is the correct designation for this field, because even now feminist therapy is not fully formed. Just as feminism is a subject in the social and political arena, and an analytical perspective to be reckoned with in the humanities and social sciences, it is also a major force in mental health. It generates

1

important understandings of personality, the practice of therapy, and methods of making change. Many aspects of the early development of feminist practice have become generally accepted elements of competent practice in today's mainstream therapy. For example, increased attention to the therapy relationship, especially in matters of power and communication between client and therapist, reflects very clearly the impact of feminist therapy. Holding clients' stories (their understanding of their experiences) as valid, and indeed central to therapy, is a heritage of feminist therapy. Informed consent and prohibitions against therapist usury—whether economic, ego-gratifying, or sexual in nature—are further changes in therapy practice wrought through feminist therapy analysis and action. Another major contribution to contemporary therapy is the influence of the sociopolitical context on the individual. Models, theories, and orientations, including multicultural, constructivist, narrative, liberation, and ecological, have been influenced by this awareness and the need to change social policy and embedded values. Feminist therapy insisted upon attending to factors affecting clients beyond the traits, personality structures, and learning patterns emphasized by earlier psychological theories (factors such as culture, race and ethnicity, gender, and class). These important changes in theory and practice have been strongly influenced by feminist therapy, albeit as in the case of other women's work, without sufficient acknowledgment.

Although many aspects of feminist therapy now central to mainstream theory and practice remain unattributed, a few have been acknowledged in the brief summaries that appear in new counseling and personality theory texts. For example, Linda Seligman's *Theories of Counseling and Psychotherapy* (2006) includes three pages on feminist therapy in a chapter with five other "Emerging Approaches Emphasizing Emotions and Sensations" (p. 244). Her brief discussion of feminist therapy mentions gender roles, self-actualization and empowerment, and feminist therapy's consistency with current trends in the field. Seligman, however, positions feminist therapy as similar to narrative and constructivist therapies. She fails to note that feminist therapy came first and influences the others. Nor is the sociopolitical influence and activist aspect presented in her cursory description of feminist therapy in this basic counseling theory text. Moreover, she misses central aspects of feminist therapy theory and practice, such as reducing power asymmetries within hierarchies, questioning the assumptions and constructs of traditional psychopathology and personality theory, and working to understand multiple oppressions experienced by women and others in nondominant status categories. Ensuring that feminist ethics explicate the harmful impact of social, cultural, and economic structures on individuals is among the foundational principles of contemporary feminist therapy. These principles lead to activism or working toward social change.

In some circles, feminist therapy is turning to action against the damaging sociostructural influence of current mental health policies and practices. The politics of mental health and the social, professional, and economic factors that support these politics are areas of current emphasis in feminist therapy.

CHANGES IN OWNERSHIP OF THERAPY

The development of therapy has taken several turns. One of these has been toward the increasing hegemonic control of therapy. Who therapy is "for" and who "owns" therapy are critical, complex, and related questions. In earlier times therapy was "for" the clients and was "owned" and controlled mutually by the client and the therapist. Perhaps 20 years ago, therapists and clients made the arrangements for therapy themselves. Although the assumption of an individual etiology for problems, interpretations that reinforced the status quo, and hierarchal decision making were certainly problems, arrangements about payment, length, direction, and interventions were all decided between client and therapist. There were three basic orientations—psychodynamic, humanistic, and radical—and a plethora of interventions to facilitate specific changes. University-based graduate programs, professional associations with ethical codes, and licensing boards existed but were separate from one another. Their roles were quite distinct and seldom overlapped. The world of independent mental health practice has changed dramatically. Today's mental health practice is no longer an independent matter of mutual decision making between clients and therapists. Instead, interlocking forces largely control the industry. Training programs, publishers, professional associations, licensing boards, and ethics committees at state and national levels control the who, what, and where of mental health practice and services. In turn, these bodies are strongly influenced by corporate economic interests.

In the 1980s medical insurance companies began to offer benefits for mental health care provided by licensed psychiatrists, psychologists, and clinical social workers. People quickly began availing themselves of these benefits, and they became very popular. However, the heavy use of these mental health benefits, combined with dramatically increasing medical care costs, led health insurance corporations to institute policy and procedural changes. Increased benefit costs, restrictions on the type and length of reimbursable treatments, pressure for lower-cost providers, and the refusal of benefits to individuals on the basis of their medical history were among the initial adjustments.

Then came the health management organizations (HMOs). These entities frequently collaborated with physicians and psychologists (e.g., in the entrepreneurial group) to initiate programs that emphasized maintaining health and that provided a set of benefits limited to the healthy. The services were more restrictive, and the premiums were lower than those of comprehensive health insurances. Quickly, HMOs became popular with employers and profitable for the corporate owners (stock in these early companies traded on Wall Street). They became the leading type of health insurance, with nearly all companies offering several policies combining different benefits and restrictions. Mental health benefits were sometimes "carved out," meaning that another corporate entity was paid a fee to manage them (i.e., to limit access to and payment for services). As corporations gained more experience, other modifications (such as limits on the number of sessions authorized, mandated clinical reviews, and clinical guidelines based on symptom reduction and strongly supporting cognitive-behavioral therapy [CBT] and psychopharmacology) were implemented.

These restrictions on payment levels, types of approved services, and length of treatment have created a situation of scarce resources, which hinders access to and utilization of mental health services. For most people, therapy is now a matter of identifying a provider on a list approved by one's insurance who has the time and expertise to treat one's particular illness or difficulty. Once a provider is found, a limited number of sessions typically are allowed to treat the diagnosed illness, according to treatment guidelines approved by the insurance company. Further, the number of providers is limited, so that a large number of patients can be guaranteed to each provider in exchange for lower payments. New or newly relocated professionals frequently have difficulty being admitted to the provider panels of insurance companies. The funding of therapy through health care insurance has led to the medicalization of therapy.

CONSEQUENCES OF CORPORATE OWNERSHIP OF THERAPY

The medicalization of mental health has affected not only individual clients, but also state licensing boards, professional organizations, and graduate training programs. Concerned for the welfare of the public, legislatures passed licensing laws for mental health practitioners and directed state licensing boards to implement the laws. Professional associations campaigned to have their own professional groups recognized by statute—an initial necessary step for third-party reimbursement. Some professional groups also worked to exclude other groups of mental health professionals. Training programs scrambled to meet the curriculum and supervision requirements dictated by these laws. National associations worked to develop, and then advocate, for licensing laws in all

50 U.S. states. Ethics boards and committees began to consider standards of care and "best practices," as defined by treatment guidelines propagated by HMOs.

Therapists engaging in unique, innovative, or nontraditional practices were vulnerable to ethics charges, which effectively barred them from provider panels and perhaps from licensure.

Because U.S. medicine has been based on the scientific method's demonstration of measurable change, this became the standard for mental health treatment and research as well. Insurance companies were quick to endorse "best practice" guidelines in mental health care, just as they had in physical health care. Guidelines for treatment of each diagnosis, largely cognitive-behavioral and pharmacological in nature, could be developed. These guidelines relied on the reduction of symptoms as the criterion for efficacy. The promises of prediction and control offered by the scientific method could thus be profitably used in mental illness, as they had in physical illness. Although the medical model and its associated diagnosis and treatment guidelines have considerable value, there are clear and important limits too.

University, hospital, and National Institute of Mental Health (NIMH) researchers have conducted and reported substantial research that develops and supports these guidelines. Some of this research has been funded by grants from corporations that sell insurance or that develop and manufacture psychiatric medications. More generally, traditional research designs require measurable variables and controlled studies, which may have debatable relevance to the concerns of real-life clients, who are very much influenced by context and who may have multiple concerns and be vulnerable to a variety of life events during the course of their therapy. Laboratory studies, carried out in an environment isolated from this real-world context, frequently fail to measure such variables as mood, sleep, and social interaction.

Training programs, unfortunately, increasingly value and rely on these research results in their course materials, supervision, examinations, and other evaluations of students' competencies. Indeed, the retention and promotion of the faculty in many programs is related to the research they have had published and the grants they have received. The textbooks used in courses are selected on the basis of contracts between the publishers and authors that center on the assurance of profitable markets for the texts.

Current efforts to control the practice of psychotherapy through science and corporate profit-making have not been successful from the perspective of individuals who have mental health needs. Their treatment has not improved, and their insurance costs have not been reduced. Cost measures implemented by managed care companies to control costs by limiting mental health access, treatment options, and duration of service have neither reduced quickly escalating health insurance costs nor provided broader access to care for citizens. Despite the clear failure of free market controls, the health care crisis in the United States has not been substantially addressed.

THE POSITION OF FEMINIST THERAPY

The economics behind today's mainstream mental health practices makes clear the politics of diagnosis and the politics of payment. "Who is therapy for?" and "Who owns therapy?" are critical and complicated questions. Analyses of power and the consideration of multiple perspectives are discussions largely absent in today's mental health literature. Both, however, are central to feminist therapy theory and practice. Feminist therapy incorporates an acute analysis of power in the therapeutic relationship and in therapy practices, including assessment, diagnosis, and the selection of goals and interventions. It also holds multiple perspectives. One of the quintessential views of feminist therapy is that socio-structural, cultural, and relational dimensions must all be considered both in conceptualization and in practice. Indeed, the appreciation of linkages among the sociostructural influences and the relational and cultural influences on the individual is one of the greatest strengths and contributions of feminist therapy, and its absence is one of the greatest weaknesses of contemporary, mainstream mental health. Individuals may be—and often are—stressed, hurt, and damaged by social events or by the effects of culturally embedded structures that limit their options. Conversely, they may be strengthened in their coping by positive aspects of their culture and by authentic, trusted relationships. Many of the clients therapists see are these types of individuals. The primary problem may be sociostructural or relational in nature, and the solution may be to engage and support cultural resources. Stress management and medication may follow, or they may be irrelevant. Keeping multiple perspectives in mind is central to feminist therapy. Yet feminist therapy is no longer alone in considering culture, race or ethnicity, economic standing, and other such categories. Several allies have come to the discussion and can be grouped together under the term "critical psychology."

ALLIED FORCES

Critical theory, as it pertains to psychology, draws together standpoints that question the underlying normative standards and values in mainstream psychology, which can be seen as contributing to injustices rather than promoting human welfare. Critical psychology is a developing area within this theory. It is informed by feminist theory, transformative multiculturalism, liberation perspectives, and postcolonial standpoints. Although these positions have their own theoretical concerns, active literatures, and practitioners, they share common theoretical underpinnings and underlying values and are important contributors to critical theory.

Like the other critical standpoints in feminist, multicultural, antiracist, and liberation theories, critical psychology shares a commitment to viewing reality from the perspectives of nondominant groups, rather than from the status quo. Fox and Prilletensky (1997), joint editors of an anthology titled *Critical Psychology*, describe the goal of critical psychologists as being "agents for social change rather than agents of social control" (p. 5). Critical theory, as it has come to community and social psychology, offers an integrative position that explicitly examines the theory, inquiry, and practices of psychology from outside of the dominant standpoint. This is especially important for groups whose experiences and history do not share equally in sociopolitical power, or in the economic and cultural structures that interlock to support the dominant group.

Gender, race or ethnicity, class, age, ability status, sexual identities, and a host of other categories are important concerns, but critical psychology's point of departure is the realization that these categories have historically been, and continue to be, used to judge one another; to place people in positions of relative worth; and to shape theory, practices, and structures into status hierarchies. Challenging the function of these status categories—and psychology's role in creating and maintaining them—is the call of critical psychology.

To the degree that we value social justice and human welfare in psychology, we must engage in a broader analysis of our constructs, methods, underlying assumptions, and practices. And we must find intellectual structures and standpoints that help us transcend the narrow, ahistorical, and largely unexamined ideological underpinnings and normative criteria of mainstream academic and professional psychology in North America.

Feminist therapy has developed its understanding of gender as inseparable from race or ethnicity, social class, and geographical region. This hard-won integrated perspective, necessary though it is, is not sufficient in the search for the power of normative structures in our society and in the theories and methods of inquiry in mainstream psychology. Gender sensitivity, cultural competence, and the challenge of the status quo are three of the supporting pillars that need to be brought to any psychology that professes to serve justice as well as healing. Both critical psychology and feminist therapy argue that without justice there is no true and effective healing. Feminist therapy theory and practice are well developed in these areas. They also place much attention on how to enact these analyses in therapeutic relationships and associated practices, including advocacy and activism. These dimensions have not yet been addressed by several of our allied, critical perspectives. Feminist therapy brings to the table of critical psychology 30 years' worth of carefully developed practice—an enactment of the principles of justice within the therapy itself. We join our allies in understanding the centrality of justice, and we lead them in its practice.

REFERENCES

Ballou, M., & Brown, L. (2002). *Rethinking mental health & disorders: Feminist perspectives.* New York: Guilford Press.

Broverman, I., Broverman, D., Clarkson, F., Rosenkrantz, P., & Vogel, S. (1970). Sex-role stereotypes and clinical judgments of mental health. *Journal of Consulting and Clinical Psychology, 34,* 1–7.

Chesler, P. (1972). *Women and madness.* Garden City, NY: Doubleday.

Fox, D., & Prilletensky, I. (1997). *Critical psychology.* London: Sage.

Mander, A., & Rush, A. (1974). *Feminism as therapy.* New York: Random House.

Seligman, L. (2006). *Theories of counseling and psychotherapy systems, strategies and skills.* Upper Saddle River, NJ: Pearson Merrill Prentice Hall.

CHAPTER 2

The Context of Therapy: *Application*

Mary Margaret Hart

Applying the principles of feminist therapy theory to the actual practice of therapy in the many diverse settings in which feminist therapists work presents a real challenge. The context in which therapy occurs affects issues such as payment, the use of diagnoses, the setting of goals, confidentiality, the power of those with whom we work both within and outside of the therapy relationship, and many other aspects of therapy. The desire for consistency between the therapist's values and theoretical framework and her practice requires a great deal—a constant awareness of the implications of behavior and decisions, a great deal of creativity and flexibility, and often courage.

This chapter presents some of the challenges that confront people who take on the work of feminist therapy. It raises some of the questions that come up when attempting to translate ideas (and ideals) into actions and also offers some thoughts about how the challenges and questions can be addressed. However, this is by no means either an exhaustive presentation or a prescription for practice. What is offered here in terms of the application of theory to practice comes as much from an increasing awareness of what isn't done consistently, of the individual therapist's limits and blind spots, as from successes in living and working as a feminist therapist. The goal of this chapter is to stimulate further thinking, and action, for each reader.

Feminist therapists face the ongoing task of challenging the often-oppressive structures of the status quo while simultaneously recognizing the concrete, specific situations and problems confronting the people with whom they are working. Both the therapist and the person in therapy live within the realities of those structures, and both are frequently faced with limited resources and options, constraining social attitudes and biases, and multiple and sometimes conflicting connections and allegiances. Therapists cannot ignore this reality and must work within it, but they also cannot afford to legitimize its oppressive elements by accommodating them easily. This social structure, with its limits and possibilities, encompasses both partners in the project of therapy, the therapist and the person in therapy. Its many facets form the context within which therapy occurs, and this chapter addresses this context, looking at the way it affects access to therapy, assessment, language and communication, the experience of power, and the therapy relationship.

ACCESS TO THERAPY IN CONTEXT

To begin with, a feminist therapist's availability, the ease with which people can initiate therapy with her, is determined by factors that go well beyond individually specific factors such as motivation, the match between the skills and needs of both people, or the compatibility of individual personalities. (The feminist therapist is referred to in this chapter as "she" or "her" to reduce awkwardness in reading. Also, although there are male therapists who work within a feminist framework, it remains true that the vast majority of feminist therapists are women.) For example, a therapist working as an employee in a community mental health agency is often unable to make the decision about whether to work with a particular individual; people do not contact the therapist directly but instead contact the agency, such as the local county mental health center. In this setting, screening for "eligibility for services" often happens without a particular therapist even becoming aware of the person's presence in the system. Also, people are usually assigned to particular therapists by supervisors or support staff. In the rural area with which I am most familiar, people are often referred to other agencies because they live outside arbitrary boundaries that determine eligibility (such as county lines) or because they don't meet other eligibility requirements. Because the county lines can divide small communities, people who could walk to one agency office but who live on the other side of this line might be required to travel 20 to 30 miles to their county mental health center, and in rural areas public transportation is either extremely limited or nonexistent. The therapist may also be aware that the therapy provided by another agency is inadequate (not to mention not feminist) but not be able to intervene, even if the person called the therapist's office or was specifically requesting to see that therapist.

The frequency and number of sessions and the type of therapy (e.g., individual, couples, or group)—and thus the scope and depth of therapy offered in an agency—is also determined at least in part by procedures and policies over which an individual therapist has little control. These in turn have been developed according to mission statements and guidelines based on worldviews that both assume and support the status quo. For instance, the medical model defines therapy as treatment and acceptable therapy goals in terms of symptom reduction and ability to function within an unchallenged social system. It also assumes many oppressive or culturally insensitive definitions of mental "health" and appropriate behavior.

Those who seek help within publicly supported mental health systems usually do not have the freedom to choose a feminist therapist; they are rarely offered information about different therapists' approaches to therapy when they choose a therapist. They may have little choice even about whether to engage in therapy because their participation may be required by those who have power to affect their lives in important ways (such as child welfare agencies, the courts, or employers who require substance abuse treatment as a condition of continued employment). For those with little money, there is usually little choice about the type of therapy they receive, or even whether therapy is offered as an option. Treatment may consist of medication and participation in diagnosis-based groups designed more to monitor treatment compliance than to provide psychotherapy. Thus, those who enter the agencies in which a feminist therapist might work come with limited control and choices both in the world outside the agency and within the agency itself.

Anna and Sergei (described in detail in the introduction), with no health insurance and severely strained finances, will probably enter the feminist therapist's small office in a community mental health center. They will probably come compelled by their fear of losing their children and their fear of being forced to return to Russia, feeling vulnerable in ways that have nothing to do with individual personalities. The therapist can't deflect the power conferred on her by these vulnerabilities by attending only to individual and relationship dynamics. The therapist's reassurances about her personal acceptance and support and her work to establish rapport are important but will have only a limited effect on Anna and Sergei's experience of powerlessness and vulnerability within therapy. At best they may feel reassured that their fate is in the hands of a benevolent but still powerful therapist, and this security is not a substitute for empowerment.

It isn't only within community mental health or other agency settings that options in choosing care are constricted by the limited availability of therapists or by the limited range of therapy offered by each therapist. For example, the therapist working with Abby (who is also described in detail in the introduction) could come to believe that the interactions provided by a safe group setting would be ideal instead of or in addition to individual therapy. Groups offer opportunities to experience shared strength and to reduce the shame associated with secrecy and isolation. This is particularly important for someone such as Abby, for whom the larger context of racial oppression will shape the meaning she gives to the sexual abuse she experienced. The power of sharing experiences is a lesson learned well by feminists (witness the often transformative effects of consciousness-raising groups in the 1970s). A feminist therapist is in the position to recognize both the larger system of oppression and Abby's individual needs within therapy.

However, the therapist may not be able to offer Abby that group experience; she may not have the time to set up a group in a busy office, and other groups may not exist. The therapist may face other obstacles, such as the difficulty of finding other potential group members who share similar experiences and who can all meet at the same time in a consistent way, a particular problem in a rural or small-town setting. It may be that any group the therapist did start would mirror the isolation that Abby would feel in the wider community; in many areas she could be the only woman of color. Although this does not mean that a group of sexual abuse survivors would not be helpful for Abby, it does mean that such a group could not provide her with the opportunity to recognize in others her own experience of dealing with this issue as a black woman in a community all too ready to see the worst in black men like her stepfather. It is also possible the therapist might not feel skilled with a group therapy format, having little opportunity to work in this way. In all these examples Abby's choices would be limited regardless of her social class or ability to pay.

A self-employed (which is not really the same as independent) therapist in private practice might seem to have more flexibility, but she still works within limits imposed by circumstances and by institutions over which she has little if any direct control. Especially significant is the increasingly intrusive and restrictive influence of health insurance companies and their use of large behavioral health managed care companies to manage cost (rather than care). Reliance on so-called third party payers has always required at least some accommodation to a nonfeminist, medical model framework, such as providing a diagnosis as a condition of payment. The accommodations required have dramatically increased over the last decades, however. The number of sessions approved for payment is now dependent not only on the presentation of a medically recognized diagnosis but also on the demonstration (to the insurance company) of the need for treatment ("medical necessity"). Demonstrating progress toward measurable goals may be required as well, especially for extended treatment or referral to "higher levels of care" such as hospitalization or intensive outpatient work. In addition, the ability to make full or even partial use of insurance coverage is often restricted by the need to see an "in-network provider."

Very few of the people with whom the feminist therapist works can afford to pay for therapy without using some insurance benefits, especially if the issues that bring them to therapy cannot be resolved in a few sessions. Most therapists make their living doing this work and are not in a position to entirely remove economic influences from the decision about whether to work with someone. Thus, both the person considering therapy and the therapist must ask themselves whether they can afford to work together. This decision must sometimes be made at several points in the process of therapy, given that many external factors can influence the availability of insurance benefits—the person may lose the job on which benefits depended; a divorce may result in a loss or change of insurance coverage; or the person's employer may change insurance carriers in order to save money, and the therapist may not be on the new company's panel. Also, changing individual or family circumstances may mean that finances are more strained, and copays that were once affordable no longer are.

These economic considerations are imposed by a social and cultural system in which care is viewed as part of the system of commerce: care becomes something an individual must purchase, and giving care is a service provided in order to meet the economic needs of the caregiver. The institutional framework within which this commerce occurs is thus motivated in large part by economics (profit-driven), is largely insensitive to individual variability (rule governed), and has little allegiance to either its "members" or the therapists it "empanels." Negotiating a way through this system so that the needs of both people involved in the therapy process are respected often requires making decisions that are at best less than ideal and at worst less than adequate for one or both people. Feminist therapists must struggle with therapy decisions that are often made for financial rather than therapeutic reasons: decisions to reduce the frequency of sessions, to limit the length of therapy and thus its scope, or to disrupt the therapy relationship by referring someone to a different therapist. These decisions are difficult and often painful, and rarely is it absolutely clear how to balance the needs of everyone involved or the therapist's own conflicting values.

For example, although Abby may enter therapy without the constraints of poverty and with middle-class resources, she may still have insurance coverage with very limited benefits for therapy, so most likely, therapy that would address fully the effects of her stepfather's molestation would have to occur at least in part without insurance coverage. All of the options open to Abby and her therapist have limitations. Focusing on managing the anxiety that Abby is currently experiencing and increasing her range of skills in this area might be possible within a limited time frame and would not be valueless. However, she will continue to have to expend energy to manage her reactions to the ongoing effects of this experience. On the other hand, committing to long-term therapy in ways that would create new problems, such as the accumulation of debt, may increase the pressure she feels in therapy and undermine the ways that therapy could offer new experiences for her.

EVALUATION, ASSESSMENT, AND DIAGNOSIS IN CONTEXT

Identifying and clarifying the problems or distress that bring a person to therapy is one of the first tasks confronting the person in therapy and the therapist. An initial assessment that is not individually focused, that defines the "presenting problems" in terms of all the systems in which they are embedded (problems *for* rather than *with* the person), can be extremely powerful in directing attention to the power of larger systems outside the therapy relationship itself. Such an "intake" is experienced as a joint project by everyone involved, a therapeutic process in itself rather than just information gathering. This in turn allows more opportunity for the person to experience the therapist as an ally and partner in a shared effort. The work becomes a shared struggle from the beginning.

Feminist concerns about the use of diagnostic codes become especially relevant during the initial assessment, but continue to apply throughout the process. The therapist's dependence on payment by third parties to make a living, either directly or indirectly (as when working for an agency that does the billing), and the person's need to use insurance benefits make the feminist therapist the point of intersection between the person seeking therapy and those who control payment. The requirement to provide a diagnosis as a condition of insurance coverage is one of the things that put the feminist therapist in the uncomfortable position of acting as one of the "gatekeepers" controlling access.

This difference between the agenda of a feminist therapist and the agenda of the institutions that control access to therapy through economic power is apparent in the way distress is defined and explained. When the individual's distress is seen as at least in part a result of an oppressive social order, the therapist is recognizing that the needs of the person and the social order are often in opposition. This is not to say that the person might not have goals that parallel this societal agenda. For instance, Abby may want to reduce the way her anxiety restricts her life, in both large and small ways. However, the motivations driving Abby differ from the motivations of organizations and institutions such as health insurance companies. Abby desires a release from fear and the power to make choices more freely. Her insurance company wants to stop paying for doctor's visits, therapy, and medications. It also wants to reduce the possibility of the need for future treatment and wants to satisfy the employer (who is its real customer) that Abby's productivity will not be threatened.

If Abby were to challenge her taken-for-granted acceptance of culturally dominant beliefs and values during the course of therapy, this could open her up to temporarily increased anxiety, to disruption in family relationships, or to redefining herself in socially unacceptable ways (for instance, if she were to become aware of and explore other options for sexual orientation in the process of dealing more directly with her own sexuality). Changes defined as unhealthy or disruptive within the context of dominant social and cultural values are likely to be viewed by third-party payers as therapy problems or failures or as unnecessarily extending treatment. In some cases, such therapy "failures" are seen as evidence that the person or the person's problems are "not appropriate for psychotherapy" or even that the person is not capable of change and is "permanently disabled." Failure to progress in ways defined by a medical model can also be seen by third-party payers as an indication that the therapist is not sufficiently skilled as a therapist or is wasting resources. This can be punished by denial of authorization for continued therapy, by a decrease in referrals, or even by exclusion from network panels.

Most people enter therapy with an unexamined and unquestioned acceptance of the social bias toward seeing problems as indications of individual deficiency or failure. For instance, Anna and Sergei may answer the therapist's question "Why are you here?" in ways that focus on their own perceived failures to manage or on personal descriptions (e.g., "I keep losing my temper"; "We can't cooperate in making decisions"; "She doesn't understand how hard I'm trying"; "I worry too much"). The therapist can open up this narrow focus by asking why they think this is happening and by asking for examples of situations or times in which they wouldn't describe themselves this way. A framework is thus established in which the problems can be defined more clearly, and the contributing factors are looked for more broadly than the small circles of these two individuals and their immediate social network.

This framework allows Anna and Sergei to name contributions to the current situation on all levels: personal experience, social relationships, institutionally imposed obstacles, and cultural norms and attitudes. They might end up talking about what makes it difficult for an immigrant to find work, the confusion of dealing with a health care system in which access is determined by the availability of health insurance, and the barriers of language to creating a system of support. Their fear of being reported to authorities can be openly discussed in terms of the power of institutions such as child welfare agencies and the immigration service. Their personal experiences growing up in a Russian cultural and historical context would inform the way they experience and make sense of all of these factors. This discussion provides a context for the therapist to ask how these things might affect the way they feel about being in therapy and what concerns they have about their therapist. Anna and Sergei might be more likely to acknowledge concerns or negative feelings openly within a discussion that includes this broader context; otherwise, their questions and answers might be constrained by feelings of vulnerability, politeness, or a desire to preserve their relationship with their therapist.

This approach to an assessment of problems and distress, rather than of people, directs the therapist, Anna, and Sergei to look at areas of their personal and shared experiences that might be outside of awareness or be so taken for granted as to become invisible. The therapist's questions would open up discussion not only of Anna's and Sergei's own personal family histories and how they perceive their different roles as parents and spouses but also of the differences they see between Russian and American values and norms and how they feel about these roles. They could become more aware of the significance of the wearing effects of Sergei's chronic pain, of the unrelenting concern they feel for their child's health, of having to constantly adapt to unfamiliar language and customs (in an environment in which others do not feel a need to also accommodate them), of not being able to assume that they are known and valued, of the suspiciousness and resentment they experience from those who see immigrants as competition for scarce resources.

This kind of assessment of the couple's problems is thus generated out of their personal experience but is not limited by an individualistic focus or a bias toward pathology. It is personal in the sense that the individual is seen as the focal point of a network of realities that together constitute the person's experience. At any given time, one aspect of experience may become the figure that stands out, but the total network of realities is always the ground that defines the experience. A feminist therapist is committed to maintaining awareness of this multiplicity and to facilitating this awareness in others. The process of assessment has to include all of these realities: physical (e.g., temperament, biologically based resiliencies and vulnerabilities), relational (e.g., personal social network, past experiences of relationships), cognitive (e.g., thinking style, language-based conceptual framework), emotional (e.g., emotional meanings attributed to events and people, self-protective reactions developed in response to past experiences), institutional (e.g., employment, legal issues, relationship to various agencies), economic (e.g., income relative to others, stability of income, degree of financial dependence, opportunities and constraints imposed by the larger economic system), and cultural (e.g., shared definitions of what is valuable, the attributes attached to different social roles, the relative emphases placed on individual autonomy and social interconnectedness). The strength of a feminist approach to therapy is that it is continually locating all of these realities within the experience of the individual. It focuses on a process of increasing awareness and change that grows out of and then beyond the individual's experience.

The feminist therapist tries to reflect this awareness of and attention to multiple contributions to a person's current experience in the written forms and questionnaires that she uses. Instead of presenting a checklist of symptoms such as mood and anxiety, forms can pose open-ended questions, asking, for instance, about the stresses and problems the person is struggling with currently, the effects these are having, and how the person has tried to manage these stresses. Opportunities to describe connections within a relational network provide a view of the person that goes beyond simplistic notions of support and isolation. Disconnection or isolation caused by relational difficulties (e.g., having conflicting goals) is experienced differently than disconnection or isolation caused by external circumstances (e.g., partners working opposite shifts with little opportunity to interact), and each would form part of the context for understanding the problems and for the therapy itself. Also, the person may not have regular contact with emotionally important people, and important people are not always supportive. The questionnaire can also inquire about connections to cultural systems, making sources of both support and alienation more visible by asking directly about racial, ethnic, or other group connections that have played an important part in the person's life. The questionnaire can also ask about other sources of emotional strength and support such as religious faith, a spiritual or intellectual practice, or a self-help program. In inquiries about health, questions can be included about the impact of past and present illnesses, injuries, and chronic health conditions. It can also be very helpful to ask how the person feels about past and present health care she or he has received or is receiving and how easy it is to communicate with those who provide care. (See the forms in Appendix A for examples of how these questions might be incorporated.)

Any discussion about the place of a "diagnosis" will then grow out of this expanded process of assessment. Because both the therapist and the person in therapy have already been engaged in developing a broad-based definition of the problem(s) facing the person, the concept of diagnosis can be introduced in a framework that is not as limited and restrictive as that which underlies diagnosis within a medical model. An explicit and multidimensional conceptualization of the problematic situation that the person is confronting can be labeled as a "working diagnosis of the problem," and thus diagnosis can be truly a guide to developing individualized (not individual) solutions. Putting this on paper, labeled "diagnosis of the problem," can be helpful (for both the therapist and the person with whom she is working) in reinforcing this reframing of diagnosis as applicable to situations and problems rather than to people.

For example, reframing the situation facing Scott and his parents (described in detail in the introduction) in a way that emphasizes the interconnectedness of many factors would be critical if the feminist therapist wanted to avoid colluding with a system that labels those who are different or devalued as problems. The family's distress might be defined as a set of interconnected parts: Scott's difficulty finding a way to be himself in a social environment that devalues some of the things he values; the parents' difficulty helping Scott transfer the values he feels free to claim and the skills he uses at home to other settings; the difficulty the school has in accommodating differences; the pervasive cultural pressure on boys to conform to stereotypical ways of behaving, which affects Scott and his peers at school in different ways.

Once diagnosis is defined in this way, the use of more restrictive diagnostic labels can be discussed. If the person in therapy is privileged enough to be free of requirements that a diagnosis be provided to insurance companies (for instance, the person is not relying on third-party payment), then a diagnostic category would be used only if it could help the therapist and the person understand an aspect of the person's situation. However, even when payment is not dependent on providing a *DSM* diagnosis, the person may be interacting with other systems in which this framework is used. For instance, when there is coordination with physicians (either primary care or psychiatrists), these labels may be imposed on whatever descriptions the therapist gives and then used as a guide to treatment. Physicians will consistently use psychiatric diagnostic codes in record keeping and in justifying decisions about treatment such as medications, and they may not be willing to prescribe antidepressants without a diagnosis of depression. Schools may require a diagnosis as a condition of providing some services. It is important for the person in therapy to have an understanding of these diagnostic labels and how they will be or could potentially be used outside the therapy relationship (for instance, in determining eligibility when a person applies for life or disability insurance).

It is also important for the feminist therapist to maintain a coherent framework within which to work, so that there is consistency in the way she conceptualizes the diagnosis (and the person in therapy) when interacting in different settings. When the therapist is required to discuss the person outside the therapy relationship with people who do not share her theoretical approach—in treatment teams and case presentations, with insurance companies, and with psychiatrists and primary care physicians—it is easy to slip into the "professional" roles and jargon that structure those institutional settings. Most professional settings maintain the convenient illusion that these socially constructed and often arbitrary diagnostic categories represent an external reality that adequately describes (or even explains) individual people. Because decisions that affect the person in therapy may be made in these professional settings and outside of any direct interaction with the person, it is important that a feminist understanding not be rendered invisible by the therapist's participation in a language that excludes it.

For example, the therapist may want to refer the person to a doctor to be evaluated for possible medical intervention such as medication. If the therapist tells the doctor she is referring this person as part of the treatment of depression, she is using professional shorthand. This saves time, may protect confidentiality in some ways (details about the person's life and situation are not revealed), and may (but may not) convey essential information the doctor would need to decide on a medical intervention. However, the therapist may also be allowing others to believe that she shares with the doctor a whole system of assumptions on which this professional language is based—or at least she is not challenging that belief directly. This set of assumptions will undoubtedly affect the interactions the person in therapy will have as this doctor's patient. Diagnosis will affect the questions the doctor asks, the assumptions the doctor makes about the nature of the problem and the patient's functioning, the way medical interventions (such as medication) are presented to the patient, and the way the success of interventions is evaluated.

LANGUAGE: REFLECTING, REINFORCING, AND CHALLENGING THE CONTEXT OF THERAPY

Any discussion of assessment highlights the way language is always embedded in the system of meanings that form the fabric of the social environment. It is impossible to isolate and avoid those social constructions that help create and maintain inequities and injustice. Within the context of these oppressive forces, the feminist therapist knows it is important to create an atmosphere in which someone can claim the therapy process in a personal way, but this is also difficult. It means fostering a relationship in which the person entering therapy experiences real power and a sense of directing the process.

Even the language often used to communicate this experience—"ownership"—reflects the nature of the larger social structure in which therapy occurs. This is a social world in which all sorts of things are owned: property, ideas, and rights to resources. It is a society of consumerism, in which ownership confers power and the ability to acquire and consume defines wealth. It is also a society that has adapted the language of commerce to therapy, in which the participants become providers and consumers, and the choices available are determined by the ability to purchase services. Although the shift away from the patriarchal language of expert professionals and passive patients has been a good one, feminist therapists have become increasingly aware of the ways this newer language of commerce can draw both therapists and the people in therapy into an equally distorted view of power in therapy. For instance, those without money have few choices and can't be "consumers" in this sense, and applying the language of marketplace to the therapy relationship obscures this.

While writing the first draft of this chapter, I became aware of how easy it is to use this language without thought—it has become so pervasive that it is taken for granted. As my awareness of and discomfort with the impact of using this language grew, I looked for an alternative to the word "client" (defined in the dictionary as a consumer). The word was initially embraced as a positive alternative to "patient." However, looking for a word that would communicate a feminist understanding of the position of the person in therapy proved frustrating; all the potential words seemed to embody some negative aspect of the dominant culture and its power imbalances. Making up a word seemed contrived, and such a word could not be used in common discourse without misunderstanding. I decided not to use a specific word at all, instead referring to "the person in therapy" when writing. The process of making this decision dramatically increased my awareness of the pervasiveness of cultural dominance in my experience as well as the power of language in my day-to-day work. Reviewing the materials I had written to use in my work showed me how often the word client is used without thought and how this shaped the ideas being communicated. Changing both those written materials and the discourse about therapy has been surprisingly difficult but also sharpens the focus as feminist therapists try to create a new framework for therapy relationships.

The consumer model of therapy also has implications for the way the thera-pist is seen: by the therapist herself, by those who might seek therapy, and by the institutions with which she must work as a therapist. As therapists are increasingly defined as people who are hired to provide services, the signifi-cance of therapy as a personal relationship is diminished or rendered invisible. Within this context, therapists can be treated as interchangeable technicians, and emotional detachment becomes the ideal stance toward a "client." "Clients" are supposed to maintain their independence and be self-sufficient, and any-thing that fosters dependency within the relationship is seen as inappropriate. Within this model there is no conceptual basis for describing or understanding authentic experiences of interdependence and connection—only a basis for building rapport and establishing therapeutic alliances as therapy techniques, or perhaps for transference and countertransference. There is also no recognition that individuals who have experienced significant neglect and who may have little experience of the trust that grows from dependable care and nurturance may need to experience dependency in ways that are both healing and safe.

Feminist therapists see the alternative to this stance as a view of therapy in which the therapist makes a personal investment in both the person and the person's goals when the two decide to enter the therapy relationship together. The therapy thus becomes "our therapy," rather than belonging to just one person in the relationship. In doing this, the therapist takes on personal respon-sibility and vulnerability, the markers of a truly mutual relationship.

Communicating this clearly is part of what allows the therapist to enter and maintain an authentic presence with the person in therapy. However, com-munity attitudes and institutional pressures often run counter to experiencing the relationship this way. Naming this personal investment early in the therapy process and reaffirming it with her choice of words throughout the process helps keep the therapist aware of the subtle pressures to conform to dominant cultural values (both external and internal). It also creates a new framework for people entering therapy, counteracting impressions and expectations based on restrictive attitudes in the larger community. The feminist therapist creates with the other person a new context for their relationship without denying the existence of the dominant context.

Providing a written description of the therapy process that includes informa-tion about the therapist's background as well as information about such issues as confidentiality, payment, expectations, ways to reach the therapist, and so on can be very useful. It can give the person a chance to review things that have been talked about without time pressure, to think of questions that might not have come up otherwise, and to orient to an experience in which full par-ticipation is an expectation. A feminist therapist will try to write in a way that reflects her belief that the person reading this will shape and define the therapy process. This helps people turn attention to defining their own goals and also helps them see the therapist as a distinct individual with a clear commitment to this shared work. (See Appendix A for a sample questionnaire and health form and for descriptive information I provide a person starting therapy.)

This process of jointly defining the experience of therapy and developing a language that allows everyone involved to maintain these definitions occurs in many ways. For instance, early in the process Abby would be asked to describe her image of what she wants from therapy, how she hopes her life will be changed by this process. Out of this would come a discussion of what working toward these goals would require from both Abby and her therapist. Abby could be asked about her expectations of therapy and of this particular therapist. This would include what she thinks therapists are able to do in general, as well as how she sees her particular therapist's strengths and limitations (for instance, how being a middle-aged white woman would affect the therapist's work with her as a young black woman). It also would include what she thinks the therapist would need to invest. The therapist can then share her own understanding of the process of therapy and make her personal expectations for herself clear. One result of this is that the therapist's investment in the process is made explicit. In a similar way both can share their understandings of what it means to be the person in therapy and discuss the expectations for Abby's role. The way differences in experience can affect therapy can be acknowledged more easily.

If Abby's expectations for her therapist are beyond what the therapist is able or willing to do, this can be discussed clearly and openly. Through this process, the therapist can model what it means to take on only appropriate responsibility and to commit only to tasks that are within a person's ability. It also makes it easier for Abby to believe that her therapist is not being drained or harmed if at some later time the therapist extends extra effort or support—"Remember, I told you I won't do or offer to do something I can't do or can't offer to do without resentment."

Language and the type of communication it structures are important in the therapist's interactions outside the therapy room as well. The therapist's relationship within therapy occurs within broader systems, including a network of "professional" relationships. As with other issues, the therapist doesn't have the option of operating completely outside this professional setting. The conceptual framework of meanings, the language, and the roles that make up this system will inevitably structure the interactions that occur within this professional system as well as between it and other systems of meanings.

To the extent that the language of the therapy professions is familiar, the therapist may be able to anticipate the meanings that other people she interacts with will use. She can try to communicate in ways that will reduce the amount of distortion of her feminist understanding of both the person and the therapy process. This requires performing some "translation" (when possible), avoiding jargon that will carry with it assumptions she doesn't share as a feminist therapist, and deliberately calling attention to information that is likely to be overlooked or ignored.

For instance, after discussing the complexities of her current situation, Abby and her therapist may decide that an antidepressant (rather than benzodiazepines) could be helpful in reducing the anxiety she feels to more tolerable levels while they work together to increase her sense of empowerment and reduce the sense of vulnerability and threat she carries from earlier experiences. When talking with Abby's physician about the use of antidepressants that are more effective with anxiety, the therapist can include information that would reduce the chances that the physician would evaluate Abby's response to medication only in terms of reduced symptoms. For instance, the therapist could indicate that reducing Abby's reliance on checking behaviors in order to maintain a sense of control may open up more conscious awareness of issues and experiences that fuel her anxiety. If the importance of having new experiences of choice and control is stressed, the physician may also be more likely to prescribe in a way that increases Abby's sense of power in the use of her medications. This may reduce the likelihood that Abby will be treated as simply having a "chemical imbalance" or that her anxiety (with its behavioral aspects) will be viewed as a personal flaw or weakness for which medication compensates. Ideally the physician can become a collaborator in Abby's process of change if the therapist communicates the importance and appropriateness of Abby's full participation in her own care. However, there is no guarantee that this will happen; many physicians (including psychiatrists) are not willing to take the time or to share power in the way required by this type of collaborative relationship (with either Abby or her therapist). In this case the therapist's role acts as a translator and intermediary between the outside system (in this case the medical system) and Abby. The differences between the physician's approach and the way Abby and her therapist are working can be discussed with Abby. She can be helped to develop strategies that allow her to use the system effectively (get a good medical evaluation and possible medications) while maintaining a sense of power and choice within these interactions. Abby and her therapist can together develop questions that Abby can take to the appointment with her doctor. She can be encouraged to take the time she needs to make decisions about complying with the doctor's recommendations rather than agreeing that she's not feeling sure simply because she can't clearly articulate the reasons for her unease.

It would also be the therapist's responsibility to be aware of the potential impact of race-based bias and discrimination in the way doctors and other outsiders use supposedly objective and neutral professional language, such as diagnostic codes. This awareness would affect the therapist's actual interactions with others and would need to be acknowledged with Abby in therapy. This discussion could help her deal more effectively with a biased system and also help her avoid internalizing this bias. In addition, it would make it more likely that Abby and her therapist would uncover the way this bias may be affecting their own work together. In these ways therapy can become a place for Abby to experience a new kind of control that comes from the recognition of personal power and the right to make choices. This would contrast with and become an alternative to her current experience of control—fearful hypervigilance, containment, and attempts to control the possibility of threats or mistakes.

POWER AS THE CONTEXT OF THERAPY

If the feminist therapist makes a commitment both to the recognition and naming of power and to changing the power dynamics imposed by oppressive systems, she needs to do this as part of an alliance with the person in therapy, or she risks duplicating the effects of that larger system. As the therapist begins work with Anna and Sergei, for instance, she needs to establish this alliance in a way that includes an open acknowledgment of the power of systems outside the therapy relationship, power that affects not only Anna and Sergei but also the therapist personally and as a therapist. The very act of naming those social structures and cultural systems begins that process. It allows the therapist to become aware of and challenge any automatic and unexamined identification she might have with this oppressive structure. The therapist can then step into a relationship with Anna and Sergei as an individual person and not just as a representative of social institutions, such as the mental health or child welfare agencies, without denying that all involved will have to deal with the power of those institutions.

Developing a broad-based assessment of problems and strengths, and doing it together as a joint project, is the beginning of establishing a therapy relationship based on mutuality and respect. Building this alliance and working within it require the feminist therapist to acknowledge openly her relative power within the larger social system and to acknowledge that she has limited ability to change that system. She also has power within the therapy relationship, even though she may be equally or more vulnerable in other areas of her life (as occurs with a lesbian therapist working with a straight woman or a man). The feminist therapist's actions have the power to affect this person in negative as well as positive ways, whether the therapist wants this power or not. For instance, if Anna and Sergei were referred by child welfare services, the therapist may have to provide reports to that agency. If so, what kind of information must be provided? How will this information be used? The primary concern of child services is the welfare of the children, but this welfare is often defined in ways that don't challenge the taken-for-granted values of the dominant social group. Information the therapist is required to provide in these reports may be structured by the outside agency in such a way as to provide only an incomplete picture of this family.

Coordinating action and sharing information with others is often important in facilitating change. Because the structure of the outside world is defined as part of the difficulties facing the person, communication and advocacy can be part of the therapy process itself and not just an addition to therapy. This position contrasts with many other approaches to therapy, which artificially distinguish between therapy and advocacy, relegating advocacy to the realm of self-help groups or case management, treating it as a less professional activity. When advocacy becomes case management, it loses its focus on system change and becomes instead a way of helping the individual function within existing systems. Many approaches to therapy recognize the need for the person in therapy to connect understanding with action. However, the need for action to be part of the therapist's role has been denied in attempts to maintain professional boundaries and contain changes within acceptable limits.

When interacting within this context, the therapist can control what she presents but not what is perceived or how it is used. Communications such as reports will still be seen through the filter of the expectations of the other person or group. The other person's need to comply with procedures and policies used within the agency or institution will also structure what is seen as relevant. Thus, what is actually taken from a feminist assessment is likely to be an incomplete and distorted version of the original assessment. When this is acknowledged, the therapist and the person in therapy create the groundwork for working together to deal with this problem confronting both of them.

In working together, Scott, his family, and the therapist could have to deal with this problem of coordinating with outside groups in several ways. For instance, if complaints from the school about Scott's behavior prompted his parents to seek therapy, it is possible that the school may want or even require (or his parents may want) communication between the school and the therapist. The therapist can talk with Scott and his parents about the benefits and potential problems involved in this communication.

The fears and hopes Scott may have about this communication are likely to be different from those of his parents, and his parents may differ in the problems they anticipate. Their concerns may also be different from the therapist's. All of these—the hoped-for positive outcomes and the fears—should ideally be identified before this communication occurs. This will allow everyone involved to make decisions both about the content of what will be shared with the school and about the way it is shared. Power is acknowledged, shared, and used within a framework of mutuality and respect.

Scott's parents may worry about Scott being labeled a problem and may want to be sure that Scott's positive qualities are recognized and nurtured by the school. They may also be concerned that his differences will make him a target of peers. Scott may be more upset that he is not being treated "fairly," that more attention is being paid to his behavior than to the behavior of the other boys. He may also worry that any attention paid to him by teachers or school staff in trying to solve the problem will lead to more teasing and harassment by the other boys. The therapist may be concerned that Scott will be defined as the problem and that the problems with the current school structures (formal and informal) will be ignored, problems such as difficulty accommodating differences and providing safety for students, a lack of awareness of the effects of teasing and bullying, and limited effective strategies for addressing these problems.

Once these issues are all on the table, the ways that they are similar and complementary can be identified. Also, the ways that they might conflict can be acknowledged, and compromises can be developed, with the underlying assumption that each person's hopes and concerns are legitimate and should be taken into account. Everyone can work to develop strategies for interacting with the school that reflect this process. For instance, Scott's worry about getting unwanted attention from teachers can be acknowledged in the report along with recommendations for ways the school can attend to teasing and bullying that will not be seen as just a reaction to Scott's situation. Other examples of teasing could be identified with Scott's help and included in the report in a way that communicates the larger scope of the problem (meeting the therapist's needs in this way as well). This deliberate inclusion of Scott's concerns as well as his knowledge of the situation might help him feel he is helping to solve the problem, thus giving him an experience of his own power that does not require him to resort to covert resistance (tripping the other boys).

The intrusions of managed care demonstrate how the power of outside societal and economic structures affects therapy. Scott's family may have insurance that requires not just a diagnosis (certainly problematic in this situation) but also the treatment reports required by managed care. These authorization requests are usually forms intended to gather information that would indicate "medical necessity" (i.e., the individual has a disorder requiring treatment), and thus the determination of need for therapy is based on diagnostic codes, a Global Assessment of Functioning (GAF) score, a list of symptoms (usually incomplete and biased), or a combination of the three. The forms may also require a listing of "measurable and achievable" goals (for the individual being treated; goals involving changing the school would not be included) and of operationalized strategies for achieving those goals. The managed care company might see appropriate goals for Scott as including the elimination of so-called acting-out behaviors such as tripping other boys and increasing the frequency of positive interactions with other boys in "masculine" activities, with the therapeutic intervention involving tracking the incidence of each with rewards being administered for "positive" change. These are the types of goals easily understood and appreciated by managed care companies. Filling out such forms is a real challenge for the feminist therapist, and this requires the same kind of effort described earlier in the discussion of the use of language and working with outside agencies or individuals.

However, managed care companies can present an even more difficult challenge because their size, the detachment of decision makers from any contact with the people involved, and their reliance on forms and highly structured communications greatly limit the opportunities the therapist has for bringing a different framework or system of meanings into the interactions. The picture presented both of the people in therapy and of the therapy itself is almost inevitably incomplete and distorted.

In order to avoid giving managed care companies the power to define the therapy process, the company's forms can be shared with the people involved (in this case Scott and his family), and strategies for filling them out can be developed collaboratively. If goals must be listed, ones can be developed that are at least not inconsistent with the broader framework being used to inform the therapy. However, the distortions that occur when important elements are left out should be acknowledged openly and explicitly. This reduces the likelihood of confusion within the therapy relationships while also increasing awareness of the operation of these larger oppressive systems. This could be helpful as a way of opening the door to awareness of the operation of similarly oppressive and restrictive systems in other areas that affect Scott and his parents, such as the problems created by school policies and rules.

A similar process can occur when working with people who are not subject to the demands of managed care insurance, but whose care is still "managed" by those paying for therapy. This would be the case for Anna and Sergei. In community mental health settings, therapists often have to justify the type of therapy as well as its frequency and duration to supervisors who need to manage costs. The requirements of demonstrating the couples' need for therapy and also of documenting progress toward specific and measurable goals (which ultimately means progress toward termination of therapy) can be even more restrictive in this setting as public funds for mental health become more and more limited. Even agencies and supervisors committed to the well-being of the people they work with face hard choices when resources are scarce and the larger society doesn't demonstrate a matching concern. In this environment not only are the people who seek help inevitably short-changed, but staff suffer also. Salaries are low, benefits are often poor, and working conditions are difficult at best. Therapists are overwhelmed by the number of people they see, and they receive inadequate support and supervision from supervisors who are also overwhelmed.

Goals within therapy must be set and worked toward in this context, structured as it is by power, both personal and institutional. A contextualized feminist assessment process will allow the person in therapy to define the problems that need to be addressed, using the therapist to help identify relevant information and sort through it. Out of this understanding the person can set goals for therapy and can discuss with the therapist how to do this within the limitations, constraints, and possibilities present in the systems in which the therapy will take place. This discussion will include ways the therapist's power as a therapist can be used in these systems, what the limits are on her ability to meet the person's needs and to advocate, how the person's own resources and power can be brought to bear, and how the person can resist oppressive elements of these systems. With Anna and Sergei, the therapist's social position and knowledge may be effectively used by everyone: the therapist may understand how to work within the system and speak the language more effectively and may be listened to because of her position, making direct advocacy useful.

THE IMPACT OF THE CONTEXT ON RELATIONSHIPS INSIDE AND OUTSIDE THERAPY

The way the therapy relationship develops and the interactions that occur between the therapist and the people with whom she works are shaped by the context in which therapy occurs. If decisions are made together, naming the forces at work both in and out of the therapy room, and with an authentic mutual relationship as a goal, the form and direction of the relationship will be determined in part by the specific issues that this larger context will force them to confront issues that can vary from one relationship to another. Within one therapy relationship, negotiating the effect of power differences based on class or race may be more central; in another, it might be that the constraints of managed care have a more powerful effect on shaping the relationship by limiting the kind of work the therapist and person in therapy do together.

One area in which the effects of social privilege and oppression become apparent is negotiating payment for therapy. Making decisions about money requires honesty from both the therapist and the person in therapy about their personal needs. For instance, when the therapist offers to reduce or waive fees for a particular person, this decision is not without implications for their therapy relationship. The feminist therapist makes an offer like this as an act of resistance to an oppressive social order rather than out of altruism. She may also see it as a reflection of her personal investment in this particular therapeutic relationship. It is important that these adjustments in fees be experienced this way by both people involved. The therapist can counteract any impulse she might have to see herself as Abby's personal benefactor or to take on the self-serving role of rescuer if she maintains awareness of this commitment to social justice. This awareness includes the recognition of the therapist's own self-interest in social resistance and change and also an acknowledgment that her participation in this particular relationship is her own choice and not something she is doing solely for the other person.

A decision to reduce or waive fees will also have effects on the person in therapy that are not determined by the therapist's intentions, feelings, or behavior, which is another reason that it must also be discussed in these broader terms. It is necessary to address the potential for feelings of obligation or shame that can arise when the therapist works for reduced fees or pro bono. It can be tempting when the therapist sits across from Abby to assume that reassurance will be enough, especially if the therapist's own experience matches the words she offers. However, one of the ways in which feminist therapy distinguishes itself from other perspectives that maintain awareness of social and cultural structures and the role of power is that the feminist therapist sees these forces at work within the experience of the individual, as lived out in the person's emotional responses, behaviors, and interactions. Thus, when they are deciding on the goals for therapy, the therapist might offer to reduce Abby's fees when her insurance coverage ends. However, the therapist would need to recognize that her intentions and behavior will be experienced by Abby within the context of her own experience of these social forces. They can't negotiate this issue in a way that is confined to intellectual understanding.

I have used something I call "time bartering" to address this issue in a way that increases awareness of the context in which I make the offer. The approach is based on the fact that both the therapist and the person in therapy are embedded in a broader context of connections that stretch over time. I start by making it explicit that I see the offer as an investment in social change as well as in the other person as an individual. I describe, in both personal and general ways, a framework in which everyone is interdependent and in which support given to one person benefits all. I often talk about some of the help and support I have received from others who did not need or require personal repayment and who saw investment in my well-being as serving their own need to create a better world and as an expression of their own values. I describe my own investment in others as my way of sharing this commitment to community with those who have supported me and also my way of passing on the fruit of their investment.

I offer this view as a statement of my personal commitment and then ask if the other person can make a similar commitment. It is most helpful to make this commitment very concrete. I explain that I have limited time and energy, and investing those resources in the person's therapy means there is less time to offer to other forms of activism for social change. I suggest drawing up an agreement in which the therapist agrees to spend time and energy working with the person in therapy, and the person in therapy in turn agrees to invest in her or his own community the same number of hours the therapist invests in their work together. The person in therapy can do this in ways that reflect her or his own values; the therapist does not determine how the hours are spent. This commitment can be met at any time in the future that the person has time and energy to share. An accounting of the time the therapist invests can be given in much the same way that a statement of fees due would be given. In this way, she and the person in therapy become partners in social change, and reducing or eliminating fees becomes a form of collaboration. However, such discussions and creative solutions do not eliminate the awareness of differences in economic status and privilege between the therapist and the person in therapy—one person can do without this money, and the other can't. These differences need to be acknowledged openly, and the therapist also needs to be aware of the possibility of future discomfort with this arrangement and other concerns about money.

The economic factors that affect the way the therapist works reflect the economic and political power structures of the larger society and, more specifically, the biases and inadequacies of the larger health care system. The feelings of shame and resentment often experienced by some within this system, as well as the sense of entitlement experienced by others, need to be recognized as a reflection of the inequalities of the broader society.

It is also true that in the process of therapy the person's relationships outside of therapy change—new ones might develop, and ongoing relationships develop in new ways—and that these changes are formed within the multidimensional context that has been described here. For example, if social isolation is identified as a problem for Anna and Sergei, the therapist and Anna and Sergei can look for ways to build a network of support that will link the couple to groups and individuals with whom they share common interests and needs. These support networks give the people in them the strength of shared experience and power. In Anna and Sergei's native country, these links would have often seemed obvious and automatic. They were based on having a large number of people who shared common experiences and history; awareness of the similarities among individual people was heightened by a broad group-based identity that could be taken for granted. In their new environment such network building is difficult because the language differences and unfamiliar social patterns highlight the differences between the couple and the surrounding community, creating a sense of isolation. However, the therapist can help them identify parts of their experience and aspects of their lives and history that they share with others. Although their new home may have a small Russian population, it undoubtedly has other immigrants who share their difficulties in creating a new life and dealing with unfamiliar institutions. These individuals may be different from the couple in many ways, with different languages and customs, but they share the immigrant experience and have many similar needs. They can provide a sense of connection and belonging that cuts across cultural differences. Organized immigrant advocacy groups can offer this too, as well as access to information and services that help immigrants navigate confusing government regulations and social institutions and support in resisting arbitrary policies and decisions.

An awareness of a context that is larger than the individual's personal network of relationships also helps the therapist understand ways that people can experience disconnection without attributing it to personal failure or a lack of interpersonal skills. In addition, this contextual framework offers a perspective for recognizing possibilities for connection when taken-for-granted links are disrupted. For instance, if participation in a community sharing a common religious faith is important to Anna and Sergei, they can be encouraged to look to local churches to meet that part of their experience, but not as a direct substitute for what they experienced in Russia. In their native country, people in this faith community would have been linked in multiple ways, including common customs, history, and other community connections. Thus, participation in a church in the United States will be a different experience. It would feel inadequate if it were directly compared to the fuller experience of their church community in Russia or if it were expected to meet the couple's broader needs for community. However, a broader perspective on community, seeing themselves as linked to many people in different ways, can do much to reduce the focus on differences and to strengthen their sense of connection based on shared experience.

Community can also stretch beyond spatial proximity given that the Internet reduces the impact of distance. The ability to find both people and information via the Internet can allow the couple to make links to communities that do not exist in their own city: Russian-language news, national resources specific to Russian immigrants, and ties to other geographically isolated people who share their cultural background. Although possession of home computers and Internet access have become new ways of dividing social classes in our society (because of limited income), local public libraries usually offer access. The inconvenience and difficulties associated with having to gain access this way can be acknowledged and assessed in terms of whether the possible gain is worth the additional effort.

All of these connections together can then become a source of strength, offering resources the couple can feel free to claim as members of multiple communities. This process of identifying allies and building a network of connections would also be helpful to Scott and his parents and to Abby. The experience of belonging to a community, of solidarity with others, is important for everyone, but especially for those identified (either by themselves or by others) with oppressed groups. It also can be an opportunity to experience power within the larger society that they do not have as individuals.

The ways that the therapy relationship intersects with outside social institutions, such as Abby's physician or Scott's school, can be opportunities for Abby and Scott to become aware that the norms imposed by these institutions are socially constructed. Part of this awareness is the knowledge that others with whom they previously may not have recognized any connection share their experiences of difficulty within this structure.

A feminist therapist can also become one of these connections, as shared goals are highlighted. Differences in experiences, culture, and social roles and position can then be acknowledged without leading to disconnection. If, for instance, Abby and her therapist define the therapy relationship as one connection among many, in which both similarities and differences can be viewed as sources of strength, then the relationship can become a model for building other connections. Both she and her therapist can maintain an awareness of the place of this relationship within the larger social framework of potential support, and the world in which she lives can be seen as offering potential resources and not just as a source of barriers, problems, and alienation.

This perspective is not intended to keep the person from becoming "dependent" on her therapist or on therapy, a position actively promoted both within the therapy professions and by insurance companies. This concern with "independence" reflects Western cultural bias. Also, the efforts of case managers to meet the person's needs outside of therapy and to promote referral to community resources such as support groups are strongly motivated by a desire to reduce costs. A feminist therapy relationship can model instead a way to depend on connection while at the same time acknowledging that the relationship cannot provide all the connections needed by the person.

The need to expand the sense of community and connection does not exist only among those who experience the disruption of cultural dislocation. Much of the alienation and isolation that is experienced by people who share a common culture results from the overemphasis on similarity and conformity that can make belonging to a group a restricting and oppressive experience. Although awareness of being different from what is socially defined as "normal" can lead to feelings of inadequacy or shame, identification with a group, even feelings of belonging, can also become a source of emotional isolation. Being able to see beyond the narrow prescriptions of any community to which an individual belongs can allow the person to recognize and respect the differences among members of that community and also to see similarities to others in communities previously defined as "outsiders" or "not like us."

This expanded vision can free the therapist and the person working with her in therapy to see in a new light the ways they both match and differ from the norms and expectations set up within the groups with which they identify. Often these norms operate without much awareness, especially for members of dominant social groups: whites of European descent, the able-bodied, and the middle class (like this author) and men and heterosexuals (not like this author). When variability among members of the same group is more clearly recognized, difference can be normalized and is less of a threat to membership in a valued group.

The isolation of being different is also reduced by the recognition of characteristics and experiences shared with others who have been seen previously as "different from me." This recognition can become a way of establishing a sense of connection across the lines of socially imposed group boundaries and leads to valuing both differences and similarities. If it is recognized that everyone is both the same as and different from others in some way, differences lose some of their power to divide. Thus, people can be encouraged to recognize their links to others who would have initially been seen as different and unavailable as sources of support, inspiration, and connection. In this process the norms they use to evaluate themselves (often negatively) can be transformed, and the oppressive power of social divisions based on differences and status can be undermined both within the individual person and in the larger society.

ALLEGIANCES TO OTHERS WITHIN THE LARGER CONTEXT

The constant inclusion of the world outside the therapy room means that the feminist therapist must also acknowledge any commitments or allegiances she has as a therapist beyond the one to the person in the therapy relationship. In every therapy relationship, there are people connected to the situation who have a stake in the process and who will affect and be affected by the people who are actually in the office. These people must be acknowledged. In working with Anna and Sergei, it would not be only the child welfare agency that has an interest in the welfare of the children. The therapist has an ethical obligation to consider and address the impact of the actions of each person in therapy on others, especially those who are dependent or vulnerable. In many instances, this concern with the welfare of those outside the therapy room is one shared by both the therapist and the person coming into therapy, and this shared commitment can further strengthen the alliance between them.

The preoccupation with individualism and competitiveness that characterizes American culture can foster a narrow focus within therapy, one based on the unexamined assumption that each person's gain is dependent on being indifferent to the welfare of others. Within this context a therapist may treat the concerns and needs of the person in the therapy room as the only valid concerns of the therapist.

The dominant values of American society overvalue the individual self over community and connection. Such a narrow view can render other people invisible or can lead to reducing them to one-dimensional caricatures or stereotypes. This is not a helpful approach, even for people who have been victimized, invalidated, or diminished by other people. Presenting therapy as concerned with only one person's welfare (rather than the person's welfare within the larger community in which others have valid needs and interests) is a distortion of what it means to validate and support the person with whom the therapist is working. It is also dishonest and can have many unintended consequences. If the therapist took this stance with Anna and Sergei, it might further alienate the couple, dismissing their value system by defining a concern with the welfare of others (such as family still in Russia) as passive or unassertive, dependent or weak, and "unhealthy."

In attempting to counteract oppressive values and social pressures, a feminist therapist may unintentionally communicate this devaluing of connection and of commitment to relationships and communities. For instance, feeling empathy for the unreasonable and oppressive pressures under which Anna and Sergei struggle, she may tend to minimize or ignore the impact of their behavior on their children. The therapist would certainly want to work with the couple to reduce inappropriate guilt, acknowledging that it is unreasonable and self-punitive to believe that they can always rise above the overwhelming demands of their situation. However, this is not the same as saying that because it isn't the parents' fault that they are so stressed, the way their children are affected does not need to be attended to. Statements that imply this, even unintentionally, present a false dichotomy between valuing the self and valuing others and are likely to be rejected by clients such as Anna and Sergei who identify strongly with their responsibilities as parents and for whom the welfare of their children is an overriding concern. They may not express this rejection openly, but it will be a potential barrier in any attempts the therapist makes to encourage self-care or to diminish inappropriate guilt.

Similarly, in strongly empathizing with Scott in his difficulties at school, it would be easy for the therapist to treat the other boys who tease and harass him as caricatures. These boys can become symbolic representations of oppressive male society rather than individual children who deserve respect and protection and who can be negatively affected by Scott's actions. The therapist needs to maintain awareness of the individual humanity of Scott's classmates and of the role of the social context in their behavior, while at the same time appreciating the reality of Scott's experience and not denying the boys' individual responsibility for their behavior. This models for Scott an alternative to both passive victimization and hostile disconnection.

For Abby, explicit acknowledgment of the complexity of human relationships would replace a position that divides the world into neat, mutually exclusive categories of good and bad people, victims and perpetrators. It would create a setting within which she can acknowledge and respect her mixed feelings about her stepfather. This in turn allows for an experience in which she can acknowledge both her own experience and his. She can then consider the well-being of both herself and her stepfather in making decisions about such things as confronting him about the abuse. This consideration does not necessarily mean that the decisions she ultimately makes must represent the needs of each equally—because some concerns outweigh others. Abby might ultimately decide to act in a way that would have a negative impact on her stepfather, but she does not have to deny all concern for him to do so.

If the therapist can maintain and communicate this broader perspective, Abby will be less likely to feel she must make all-or-nothing choices. Anything that implies that the therapist is interested *only* in Abby's well-being or that the therapist has no concern for anyone except Abby would reinforce the assumption that there are only two options open to Abby and her therapist. Abby can easily come to feel that her own attachment to and love for her stepfather are necessarily incompatible with self-care. She might feel that she has to make a choice between herself (by rejecting her stepfather completely and denying a part of her own experience) and the relationship with her stepfather (thus devaluing or dismissing her own pain and anger—for instance, feeling her own experience "doesn't count" if he isn't a "bad" person). The recognition of the complexity of other people and of human relationships is inherently linked to the ability to recognize and value the complexity of her experience and needs.

This perspective takes in the broader context of an individual's life, seeing Abby embedded in complex relationships. However, this doesn't mean that the therapist is neutral about Abby's stepfather's actions or about the effects of those actions on Abby, only that the relationship between Abby and her stepfather cannot be reduced to just those actions. Abby's acknowledgment of those effects (and the feelings of hurt and betrayal that accompany that recognition) may change her relationship with her stepfather in profound ways. Negative effects on her stepfather can still be viewed as the consequence of *his* behavior without necessarily ignoring other experiences they share. The therapist can model and create the opportunity for Abby to take herself and all of her experience seriously. This in turn allows for self-care that is not based on a denial of parts of her experience or on a denial of the humanity of her stepfather.

CONCLUSION

All of the examples used in this chapter could be approached in different ways by different feminist therapists. The constant awareness of the context in which all individuals live out their lives and within which therapy occurs is one of the ties that unite the variety of approaches within a feminist worldview. This awareness does not ever view the individual in isolation, as if all relevant information were contained within the boundaries of each individual's biology or experience. At the same time, the individual person is not reduced to a collection of social roles or categories as if the therapist could adequately know this person at this time in this relationship by understanding the nature of social, cultural, and economic forces alone.

Instead, the person in therapy, the therapist, and the therapy relationship are seen and experienced as both embedded in and encompassing a vibrant whole under constant pressure and in constant flux. Therapy is part of this larger process, the intersection of two people's lives in this particular place and at this particular time to engage in the joint task of directing change.

A feminist therapist must live in the tension between individual experience and the broader context within which it occurs. The focus of attention may rest on different aspects at different moments, but the dynamic energy created by this tension does not allow one aspect or one moment to "stand still." This is the underlying root of the enduring principle of feminism—the personal is the political, and the political is the personal. Feminist therapy is an opportunity to recognize and validate this principle. Each time the person in therapy and the therapist become aware of this dynamic reality and then act on that awareness, each time both refuse to settle for simplistic partial truths or prescribed solutions, they engage in an act of both resistance and hope.

CHAPTER 3

The Person of the Client: *Theory*

Susan Barrett and Mary Ballou

As therapists, our beliefs about people, their personalities, and their behavior are formed largely by cultural and social expectations. These beliefs arise out of living in the larger culture, but also through our professional training. Personality theory and standards of psychopathology as learned in our training are not independent of the professional culture and broader social norms. As individual mental health professionals, we have often examined our beliefs, identifying those that are socially constructed, those that are idiosyncratic to ourselves, and those that stem from our professional training. Also, much feminist and critical mental health theory has supported this task and has called for theory that is less tied to the social norms and ruling ideologies of a specific historical period.

So although warnings about the bias and dangers of unthinking application of mainstream personality theory and standards of psychopathology have been loud and consistent, alternative views have been slower to develop and more muted. This chapter tries to address this need. It offers a way to assess and conceptualize the influences on the development of a person.

Therapy is about people, and the therapy setting is about therapists and clients in very intimate, face-to-face interactions. A major leap forward in the conceptualization of the people in therapy occurred in the 1970s, with a focus on the sex and gender of the client and the therapist. This was a radical departure from the dominant framework of male as norm. Embedded within the larger wave of that phase of the women's movement, theorizing was based on the actual experiences of women and included the influence of the culture and environment as well as more traditional psychological theory. *The Handbook of Feminist Therapy* (Rosewater & Walker, 1985) was a groundbreaking text in understanding women in therapy through the lens of sex and gender.

As important as considering the sex and gender of client and therapist is, that particular lens, taken in isolation, also has major limitations. Much of the initial theorizing of the Feminist Therapy Institute was done primarily by white professional women writing about other white middle-class women, both heterosexual and lesbian. Across the past two decades, understanding of both the client and the therapist has become far more complex.

Many women have contributed to describing and understanding this complexity, some through telling their stories and some through conceptualizing, or making sense, out of the stories they have heard and lived themselves. The experiential base of women's lives remains central to this complexity, allowing feminist therapy to draw from and interweave with literature, nonfiction, sociology, racial and cultural analyses, art and music, and many other forms of communicating about the essence of our lives.

A major aspect of this experiential base for theorizing has continued to be the effect of the current culture and environment on women. We have far more information available, in a large part because of increased access to publication, about the impact of the lived experience of a wide range of women's lives. Many psychologists and psychotherapists have written extensively about the intersection of race, class, and culture with sex and gender. Beverly Greene (1997), Lillian Comas-Diaz (2000), Oliva Espin (1999), Jean Lau Chin (2000), Maria P. P. Root (1990), Jeanne Adleman and Gloria Enguidanos (1995), and others have eloquently and persuasively both described the lives of women and developed theoretical frames for understanding those lives. Sexual identity and orientation theorizing, though still addressing the impact of minority status, has expanded to a wider range of experiences, including parenting (Clunis & Green, 2003; Martin, 1993) and transgender and non-gender identities.

Some women have examined the impact of trauma on the lives of a wide range of women, often examining the effects of trauma from perspectives that include race, class, culture, immigration status, and sexual identity (Espin, 1999; Herman, 1992; Root, 1992). One consequence of this theorizing is the realization of how pervasive trauma is in our society and how much women suffer under both chronic and acute forms of trauma. A more recent development is understanding people from the perspective of resilience, an interesting topic to pursue from a feminist viewpoint.

Other feminist psychological theorists have used the experiential base of women's lives to posit new theoretical perspectives for understanding people. Kaschak (1992) puts forth an extensive understanding of the social construction of women's lives and the psychological impact of that construction. The scholars at the Stone Center (Jordan, Walker, & Hartling, 2004; Miller, 1987) recentered Western psychological thinking away from independence and autonomy as the center pins of psychological growth and to relation and connection as the center of growth. Their work interwove with that of women ranging from Gilligan (1982) to Belenky, Clinchy, Goldberger, and Tarule (1986), who strove to articulate the importance of connection. Now we are developing the intersection of the theorizing of these white professional women with the writings of women of color, non Euro-American women, immigrant women, and others for whom connection has always provided a major way to understand their lives.

Parallel to the development of feminist therapy theory has been the development of other theoretical models based, in part, on the lived experiences of particular populations of people. Multicultural psychological theory (Sue & Sue, 2003); queer theory (Fox, 1995); theory about the effects of immigration (Javed, 1995); and ability/disability theory (Olkin, 2005), as well as the influence on individuals of specific cultural backgrounds, are examples of the multiplicity of ideas being developed that either counter or build on traditional psychological theory. All of the particular standpoints of an individual person continue to be extremely relevant, including sex and gender as addressed in feminist therapy.

At this time, a feminist understanding of how to think about the two or more people in the therapy room can benefit from this explosion of available information. On the other hand, all the information needs to be presented in a way that is useful to the therapists and to the clients. Our integrated model is one way to organize the information so that it can be useful with a wide range of therapeutic approaches. For some people, a perspective of healing, with concomitant diagnosis, is indeed relevant. For example, understanding a client as suffering from posttraumatic stress disorder (PTSD) can help both the client and the therapist understand what has happened to the client and what might be helpful for the client at this point. Many other clients come to therapy in a state of distress, such as from a relationship breakup or other life transition, and seek relief from the misery they are currently experiencing. They may not need or want a medical diagnosis. Assessing resilience, or the ability to recover from situations, may be an important part of therapy for both those needing healing and those needing relief from distress.

Yet other individuals coming to therapy don't fit these descriptions. They are coming to expand, to develop, and to become more full human beings in their own terms. None of us develop all of our psychological relational capacities. We are all influenced and limited by our particular circumstances, starting in childhood and continuing as we live our adult lives. Particularly as our population lives longer, adult growth and development becomes ever more important to understand, assess, and focus on in therapy. Regardless of whether a framework of disease and healing; relief from distress; resilience, growth, and development; or a combination of these is most relevant, the therapist needs to be able to place the client, and herself, in a contextual perspective that facilitates making sense of the current situation for the client.

Many psychological models emphasize either theory or practice, for example, focusing on information about the psychological status of varying groups of people or about how to utilize a particular form of therapy. Across the decades, feminist therapy has directly addressed both theory and practice with particular attention paid overtly to the application of theory to therapy practice. The image of a tapestry can help us translate these models into the therapy setting without the scope of the description and analysis needed becoming overwhelming. If an individual is viewed as a rich and complex tapestry, a full range of factors and threads combine to become the whole. It is essential to see the individual as the full tapestry, to hold the full range of possibilities in our minds, while focusing on certain aspects of the whole at any given point in time. We could imagine attending to one section of the total, such as a change in physical health (e.g., colon cancer). That section would include a client's individual self, her feelings, beliefs, and pain as well as her relationships with others. She might find herself in categories of group identity, that of cancer patients or of those who become disabled. She may need to learn more about communicating across group identities. All of this would also be influenced by the larger factors, such as access to resources and the structure of health care.

Another way to view the tapestry idea is to consider that, at a particular time, the client is pulling up certain threads that cut across many sections of the tapestry. For example, an individual who has defined herself as independent and autonomous may find herself yearning for connection. Pulling up the threads related to connection would cut across her individual sense of self, causing her to begin to see herself as needy as well as strong. She would need to identify how she enters into relationships, to whom is she attached, and where she finds a sense of support and holding from others. All of this is affected by a group identity—for example, some cultural and religious groups may privilege a self-contained individualistic stoicism, while others may value the power to be found in connection, mutuality, and the recognition of vulnerability. The institutional forces reinforcing independence or the planetary conditions creating natural disasters in which independence and dependence are played out are also relevant to the whole.

As therapists, the tapestry image applies to us as well. However, we also need to attend to the threads in the background that are not being addressed by the client at the moment. In other words, we need to listen to what is not being said as well as what is. Is the client attending to her or his individual experience and not seeing how that experience is common to a particular group of people, such as immigrants? Does she or he see the problem as relational in nature—if her or his partner would only be different, the person would not be in the pain she or he currently experiences? Perhaps focusing on her or his individual feelings and self care is what really would be most helpful to the person before attempting to bring that vulnerability into a relationship.

What threads, as therapists, do we see that are simply not okay to live with? How do we, as therapists, address self-injury, substance abuse, and physical, emotional, and sexual abuse of others? Even if those threads seem, to the client, to be consistent with and okay with her or his identity, how do we view them with regard to the overall tapestry of the individual?

THE INTEGRATED MODEL

We have blended two conceptual models into one integrated one as a way of organizing the information and applying it directly to the therapy setting. The original models are Barrett's (1998) model of contextual identity and Ballou, Matsumoto, and Wagner's (2002) feminist ecological model. The drawing represents the integrated model.

CONTEXTUAL IDENTITY

Because we are addressing the assessment of client and therapist within the therapy setting, the starting point of conceptualization is the lived experience of the client and the therapist as represented in the innermost ring of the drawing in Figure 3.1. Contextual identity is a complex understanding of oneself that is multifaceted and fluid, based on both individual and societal determinants that may be static or vary and evolve across time. The lived experience of an individual provides an internalized sense of self, both conscious and unconscious, a sense of who the person is and how the person understands her- or himself. This complex sense of self has four aspects and

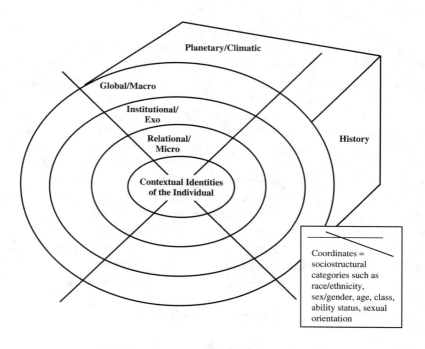

Universal
• Qualities and phenomena common to all

Global/Macro
• Political/economic
• Environmental
• Distribution of resources
• Values
• Worldviews
• Ideologies

Institutional/Exo—Regional, State, National
• Educational/political systems and structures
• Social institutions
• Legal/political systems
• Professional/disciplines
• Religion

Relational/Micro—Immediate face-to-face interactions and influences
• Family
• School
• Work
• Church
• Neighborhood

Contextual Identities of the Individual—Internalized identities of the individual person
Individual (e.g., biological, emotional, cognitive, spiritual, intuitive/creative)
Relational
Group
Universal

Figure 3.1 Contextual ecological feminist model.

carries within it the understanding that, at any specific time, a given aspect is more important than others and that each individual ascribes meaning that helps create that importance.

One aspect of identity is that of the individual. This includes a variety of personality patterns and interests that stay remarkably stable across time, such as introversion or extroversion. In addition, our individual identity includes shifts and changes that occur across time, including developmental shifts. For example, how I understand myself regarding my physical abilities and challenges is not the same at age 20 as at age 50. Other changes in individual identity are the consequence of learning and of both good and bad life experiences that alter our sense of ourselves. The individual self is biological, emotional, and cognitive, so this level of identity includes transient aspects, including our feelings, thoughts, wishes, beliefs, and other intangible and changeable understandings. Many people enter into therapy to address this individual level—for instance, to deal with pain and loss, to ease life transitions, or to find a focus for their lives. Western traditional psychotherapy has heavily emphasized this individual level of each person.

A second aspect of identity is relational: Who am I in relation to others? Who are the people I consider family and friends? How adept am I in my capacities for connecting with others? As with individual identity, this level is both stable across time and fluid and changing. Most of us have a relational identity as a son or daughter of parents, even if the parents are no longer living. We often retain an identity as a sister or brother, as a cousin or niece, even if estranged from those people. Across time, we usually add other relational identities, adding and dropping friends, creating and recreating families. Some people become parents themselves, a relational identity that often alters other ones, such as a son or daughter. Given a conflict between roles, do I act as the dutiful child or as the caring mother? Relational identity is both generic (i.e., I belong to the category of people labeled mother) and, at the same time, very particular (i.e., I am the mother of this particular child).

Relational identity has been the focus of several different groups of therapists. Marriage and family therapists often have this identity as the central focus of their work and have developed theoretical understandings and practices within which to work. The work by the theorists at the Stone Center at Wellesley College is based on the assumption of the primacy of relational needs for individuals. Josselson (1996), for example, describes in great detail several of the many important ways of being in relation to others. The theoretical work of these and others provide insight and direction for therapists as clients come to them with their yearning for connection, with the pain of relationships ending, and with the desire for help in untangling distressing knots in the connections with those they love.

A third aspect of identity, beyond the first two personal aspects, is a sense of self based on larger social units, such as race, class, and country. This level of identity includes the group identities an individual claims as well as those ascribed to her or him by others. Both internalization and ascription of group identity have an impact on a given individual, as can be seen during the process of learning to value oneself. Valuing oneself on the basis of roles or group identities valued by society (e.g., white, heterosexual, or able-bodied) is a very different experience from learning to value oneself with regard to group identities that are devalued (e.g., person of color, bisexual, or disabled). To add to the complexity, many people have group identities that are a combination of valued and devalued. Interactions of group identities with individual identities are quite complex and have not been a central concern of traditional psychotherapy.

Traditional psychotherapy has not been concerned with integrating multiple group identities with individual identity. However, as mentioned earlier, this integration has been the focus of psychological theory as it addresses particular groups.

Finally, we have a common, universal identity as human beings that transcends our differences. Physiologically and anatomically, we clearly share aspects of our selves with all other people and with no other species. And though most of us might use a concept of the universal human in our therapeutic work, just what psychological characteristics we actually share with all others has been so heavily influenced by the thinking of those in dominant groups that what is truly universal is far from clear. Frequently, an appeal to the common bond of being human is used to skip over and minimize the differences among us, particularly on the level of group identity.

All these aspects of contextual identity form the lived experience of an individual person as she or he is represented in the innermost circle of the diagram. This is a markedly expanded sense of an individual, beyond traditional psychology's understanding of a separate self. At the same time, the picture of the individual is incomplete without a way to consider all the multiple factors and layers that interact with, create, modify, or impinge on that given person. The rest of the diagram depicts these forces and is drawn from the feminist ecological model.

MICROSYSTEM

The first layer of influence is the microsystem, which encompasses the individual's immediate environment. This includes face-to-face interactions and influences that are encountered by the individual frequently—for example, relationships with family and friends, neighbors and mentors, and school and work colleagues, as well as interactions in community groups (e.g., YMCA, country clubs, or gangs), neighborhoods, local government, schools, churches, and employment settings. These relationships and structures are very important to the development of a person's beliefs and expectations. The interaction between individual cognitive, emotional, and spiritual spheres and beliefs and expectations held by those in the microsystem are central to development. These social and familial forces provide the framework for a person's expectations and normative values. A critical component of this level is the recognition that a person's values and worldview are strongly influenced by the social and political views to which the person is exposed. Exploration and questioning of these influences is imperative. If, for example, one's church community advocates for traditional sex roles that privilege men, then egalitarian relationships are not likely to be found or aspired to by these men and women.

EXOSYSTEM

The exosystem is a level of more formal organizations and social policy. Legal, governmental, educational, religious, professional, and academic disciplines set standards and make policy, thus exerting influence. These institutions claim that their rules and guidelines are fair and in the best interest of the public or their constituents, yet the policies often are made by those who have achieved status within the institutions, giving tremendous power to the rule makers. Too often these rule makers have had limited exposure to diverse experiences and situations, leading to rules and guidelines that favor one set of experiences over many others. Although it is important for people to be clear about the standards and influence at this level, interactive influence here is generally the result of activist collaborations among the disciplines and professionals. In therapy we need to understand institutional influence and power and see it as affecting us and our evaluations of our identities and experiences; however, change requires activism and collaborative efforts among disciplines, professional organizations, and affected groups. An example is the efforts to root out racism from government, religion, professional groups, and the culture at large. The hegemonic links among the rule makers within social institutions create the very real danger of normative standards that authorize one way instead of acknowledging and supporting many ways.

MACROSYSTEM

The next level of influence is the macrosystem. Here we take a broad, often global view to understand how wide-ranging systems, ideologies, and social causes (e.g., distribution of resources, advanced capitalism, technological development, global trade, nationalism, fundamentalism, and movements for social justice and human rights) are interrelated and affect us all. These macrosystem geopolitical processes directly or subtly influence each of the levels of the model. For instance, there are complex relationships among advanced capitalism, the European Economic Community (EEC), multiculturalism, and heightened tension with immigration. These have in turn fueled nationalism and fundamentalism and an increased concern about "terrorist threats," resulting in such violations of social justice as the Patriot Act and a decrease in civil liberties in the United States.

These macro forces and processes not only are at work at the broad structural level, but also extend their impact on each level of the model. Structural inequities and social injustice result in large measure from valorizing one political, economic, or religious system. The macro forces also influence expectations and standards in more local social and family groups as well as living and psychological problems. The idea that "the personal is political, and the political is personal" is a far more complicated and meaningful statement than understood at its origin. Understanding the interlocking hegemonic relationships is critical for understanding the profound pressures and frequent damage wrought by single privileged views of right, holy, best, or successful.

OTHER REALITIES

In addition to these levels, planetary conditions and the historical period are realities that affect all levels. For example, global warming, overuse of natural resources such as oil and coal, and pollution of earth, air, and sea are likely affecting our climate, worsening natural disasters, and contributing to the environmental causes of disease. In geopolitical environments, advanced capitalism and Middle Eastern oil supplies are influencing further unequal distributions of wealth nationally as well as contributing to distant economic and ideological differences between global countries.

COORDINATES

The last aspect of the model includes factors such as age, sex and gender, social and economic class, and race and ethnicity, here called coordinates. On the drawing, the coordinates are shown but not named, given that they can and do change. These socially defined and differentially evaluated constructs, attributes, and characteristics are very significant in how an individual is treated, given status, and evaluated within each of the levels. Individuals also interpret themselves and others through these coordinates. These factors are markers of dominance and nondominance, best or worst, good or bad. As much as we may want to believe in the myth of equality or meritocracy, our present systems do not reflect these values. To be male, Caucasian, upper-class, affluent, and middle-aged are the coordinates of privilege. These people are the holders of the normative standards and are the rule makers. These coordinates affect and interact with each level—on the individual level; in the immediate environment; in the institutionalization of rules and standards in social, legal, and professional systems; and in the geopolitical realm as well. These coordinates are very important because the many influencing factors of the model affect individuals differentially not only on the basis of the individual's characteristics but also according to a person's age, race or ethnicity, sex or gender, and class.

EXAMPLES OF APPLICATION OF THEORY TO PRACTICE

This integrated model offers useful ways to conceptualize matters of influence on people and their internal identities. In the following paragraphs we offer a few brief illustrations of the complex interactions among factors and identities.

- The historical event of African people being kidnapped from their homelands and sold into slavery forms an important basis for understanding the disrespect, dehumanizing treatment, and damage it has brought to African Americans. Merely identifying the social construction of race is not enough. The politics of slavery and the geopolitical effects of industrialization are important past influences on the experiences and identity of African Americans. Some of the struggles, accomplishments, and goals of African Americas today, including attribution by shade of skin, family networks, self-hate, importance of education, and inadequate public resources supporting equal educational opportunities, are related to slavery.
- The importance of planetary conditions can easily be seen in the increases in the rates of some cancers and asthma resulting from the interaction of human biology and the contamination of the physical environment caused by individual consumption and by corporations profiting through capitalism. Mothers dying, children ill and lacking good medical resources, and men desperate and disconnected because their best efforts cannot help—the plights of all these people are linked to planetary conditions as well as class- and economic resources.

- Geopolitical issues ensuing from clashes of religious, national, and ethnic groups engender the anxiety, hyper-stress, and hedonism that have become pervasive mental health problems.
- The coordinates within the ecological model are equally importantly tied to identities. Differential treatments such as fewer rights for children, less respect toward old women, and emasculation of men past their years of productive labor are all related to the interactions of age and gender. If race and ethnicity are added, the discrimination becomes even more complex when there is a depressed elder in the counseling room.
- The lack of stable sustainable communities—schools, neighborhoods, families, and even professional groups—clearly impacts the identities of today's adolescents, and this lack is likely a significant factor in adolescents' searching for connection and positive evaluation through such means as attaining an "acceptable" body size, acquiring trendy clothing, and engaging in multiple sexual encounters.

An example of the effects of these structural forces on a particular client or therapist is how these forces exert an impact on the group identity of a person and on the ability of an individual to shift between individual and group identity. The development of minority group identity, including multiple identities, stages of identity development, and fluid identities, has been the focus of many theorists, including Root (1990); Helms (1990); Sellers et al. (1998); Barrett (1990); Ahn, Suyemoto, and Carter (in press); and Prescott (2006) as well as others. Dominant group identity development, including identity built on being a member of a dominant group as well as identity built on understanding the privilege of that dominant identity, continues to be described by Helms (1990) and others.

With regard to group identity, individuals need to be able to shift between individual identity and minority and dominant group identity and to be able to communicate effectively across group identities. An inability to shift between group identity and individual identity can leave minority individuals at risk in one of two ways. They can over-personalize the prejudice coming toward them, absorbing the negative result of that; or they can minimize their personal responsibility, attribute what happens to them to their minority status, and feel victimized. Members of dominant groups who cannot shift between individual and dominant group identities are at risk of continuing to reinforce their dominance over others and also of confounding the particular with the universal. That is, they are at risk of assuming their way is the right and only way. They are also at risk of assuming that the benefits that come their way are the result of their individual effort, rather than the result of belonging to a dominant group.

The Person of the Client: *Theory*   51

As therapists, we have not routinely focused on integrating group identity with individual and relational identity. Yet the problem may be with the system, not with the individual person. A classic example is the individual struggling to come out as a lesbian, feeling isolated, numbing her feelings with alcohol, and being emotionally constricted. The individual level of distress will be difficult to address without concomitantly addressing the need to value oneself, even as microsystems and exosystems (society at small and large) devalue all but one sexual identity.

These examples show the relevance of thinking broadly and in multiple dimensions in order to apprehend the influences and interactions that are important to the composition of identities. Again, the idea is to think contextually and broadly and then, in therapy, to respond individually to that particular client.

IMPLICATIONS AND USEFULNESS OF THE INTEGRATED MODEL

This integrated model offers a powerful representation of contemporary feminist thinking, combining the influences of the structural position and personal experience in quite useful ways. The goal is to "think contextually; act personally." The model emphasizes the importance of lived experience as a central base for understanding both the client and the therapist. The importance of lived experience is represented by recognizing the multiplicity and complexity of influences and experiences for any individual. As therapists, we need to remain complex in our thinking, rather than reducing ourselves and clients to easy categories for ease and control. All African American mothers are not heterosexual or Democrat, for example. Objective information is important, but the subjective meaning an individual gives to the more factual information is the most crucial to understand. Of all these factors and influences, what is most important to a client at a given time? How is the client weighing various identities? How does the therapist understand these aspects of the client, and of herself? How does she understand the weighing a client gives to one aspect of the client's identity versus another?

Embedded in these models is the concept of pluralism, meaning equally valued difference. Hope Landrine (1995), Carol Travis (1992), and others have engaged this question of difference, similarities, and deviation in significant ways. Instead of conceptualizing difference as a deviation from a given norm that assumes one way is the right or best, *difference can be best understood as an equally important and valid way to be.* For example, holding a biracial identity is different from holding a monoracial identity. There is no better or worse, no deviation from a mean that then becomes the expected standard. Yet it is also important to point out that certain standards or ways are concordant with the dominant group's expectations, modes of functioning, and rewards systems. So although differing ways may be of equal value, the mainstream does not judge, reward, or esteem them similarly, thus the term "status categories." Heterosexuality is the mainstream standard, and although it is not better, it is valued and rewarded more than homosexuality and bisexuality.

At the same time that the models allow for pluralism, embedded in the assumptions of understanding the complexity of both the therapist and the client is the necessity for the therapist to accept responsibility for what she believes is not appropriate behavior, regardless of the particular cultural context. Kegan in *In Over Our Heads* (1998), describes the necessity of developing our own sense of moral judgments, for example, when we do not accept the models presented. If we do not accept the dominant culture's view of, for example, a good mother, we are responsible for knowing what a good mother is like and what is really not okay, such as sexual and physical abuse of children, regardless of the culture. Feminist therapy ethics combined with feminist understandings about parenting are helpful frameworks for identifying what is good and what is not.

Yet another valuable aspect of this model is its usefulness for social change. Because assessment of the client is completely embedded within the context of the person, all the multiple dimensions of the feminist ecological model must be assessed along with the identities of the client. The context within which an individual lives, rather than the identities of the person, might actually be the problem. Although attention to the client's identities would be prominent in therapy, awareness of the external influences and evaluations is also central to assessment. Not only does such assessment help clients to see the results of dominant and minority power differences; it also directs attention toward social change.

SUMMARY

The expanding understandings through integration of the two models in this chapter require more complex and multiple thinking. Current feminist and critical psychology informs therapy thinking in very important ways. As with the tapestry, the complexity is richer and more useful than mainstream assessment of individual problems. At the same time, the model, through a focus on identity, provides a clear link to therapy not necessarily addressed in models more focused on psychology than therapy. Individuals' experiences, be they developmental struggles, problems, crises, or challenges, have relational-cultural, sociostructural, and geopolitical elements. The feminist ecological model is a useful way to hear and consider these; yet where these factors touch individuals, the identities model captures the experience. The person in context and the complexities of assessment as felt in contemporary feminist therapy theory and practice are synonymous with more socially activist–oriented statements, such as "think globally; act locally." The equivalent here, as noted earlier, would be "think contextually; act personally." This chapter has discussed the integrated Barrett and Ballou models as useful in doing so. The next chapter looks at how this might be done in some detail within specific cases.

REFERENCES

Adleman, J., & Enguidanos, G. (1995). *Racism in the lives of women: Testimony, theory and guides to antiracist practice.* Binghamton, NY: Harrington Park Press.

Ahn, A. J., Suyemoto, K., & Carter, A. (in press). Relationship between physical appearance, sense of belonging, feelings of exclusion, and racial/ethnic self-identification among multiracial Japanese-European Americans. *Cultural Diversity and Ethnic Minority Psychology.*

Baker, M. J. (1987). *Toward a new psychology of women* (2nd ed.). Boston: Beacon Press.

Ballou, M., Matsumoto, A., & Wagner, M. (2002). Toward a feminist ecological theory of human nature: Theory building in response to real-world dynamics. In M. Ballou & L. Brown (Eds.), *Rethinking mental health and disorder* (pp. 99–141). New York: Guilford Press.

Barrett, S. (1990). Paths toward diversity: An intrapsychic perspective. In L. Brown & M. Root (Eds.), *Diversity and complexity in feminist therapy* (pp. 41–52). Binghamton, NY: Harrington Park Press.

Barrett, S. (1998). Contextual identity: A model for therapy and social change. In M. Hill (Ed.), *Feminist therapy as a political act* (pp 51–64). Binghamton, NY: Harrington Park Press.

Belenky, M., Clinchy, B., Goldberger, N., & Tarule, J. (1986). *Women's ways of knowing.* New York: Basic Books.

Chin, J. L. (Ed.). (2000). *Relationships among Asian American women.* Washington, DC: American Psychological Association.

Clunis, D., & Green, G. D. (2003). *The lesbian parenting book: A guide to creating families and raising children.* New York: Seal Press.

Comas-Diaz, L. (2000). An ethnopolitical approach to working with people of color. *American Psychologist, 55,* 1319–1325.

Espin, O. M. (1999). *Women crossing boundaries: A psychology of immigration and the transformation of sexuality.* New York: Routledge.

Fox, R. (1995). Bisexual identities. In A. R. D'Augelli & C. J. Patterson (Eds.), *Lesbian, gay and bisexual identities over the lifespan* (pp. 262–290). New York: Oxford University Press.

Gilligan, C. (1982). *In a different voice.* Cambridge, MA: Harvard University Press.

Greene, B. (1997). Lesbian women of color: Triple jeopardy. *Journal of Lesbian Studies: Classics in Lesbian Studies, 1,* 49–60.

Helms, J. (1990). *Black and white racial identity: Theory, research, and practice.* Westport, CT: Greenwood Press.

Herman, J. L. (1992). *Trauma and recovery* (Rev. ed.). New York: Basic Books.

Javed, N. S. (1995). Salience of loss and marginality: Life themes of "immigrant women of color" in Canada. In J. Adleman & G. Enguidanos (Eds.), *Racism in the lives of women* (pp. 13–22). Binghamton, NY: Harrington Park Press.

Jordan, J., Walker, M., & Hartling, L. (Eds.). (2004). *The complexity of connection: Writings from the Stone Center's Jean Baker Miller Training Institute.* New York: Guilford Press.

Josselson, R. (1996). *The space between us.* Thousand Oaks, CA: Sage.

Kaschak, E. (1992). *Engendered lives: A new psychology of women's experience.* New York: Basic Books.

Kegan, R. (1998). *In over our heads: The mental demands of modern life.* Cambridge, MA: Harvard University Press.

Landrine, H. (1995). Introduction: Cultural diversity, contextualism, and feminist psychology. In H. Landrine (Ed.), *Bringing cultural diversity to feminist psychology: Theory, research and practice* (pp. 1–20). Washington, DC: American Psychological Association.

Martin, A. (1993). *The lesbian and gay parenting handbook.* New York: HarperCollins.

Miller, J. B. (1987). *Toward a new psychology of women* (2nd ed.). Boston: Beacon Press.

Olkin, R. (2005). Women with disabilities. In J. C. Chrisler, C. Golden, & P. D. Rosee (Eds.), *Lectures on the psychology of women* (3rd ed.). New York: McGraw-Hill.

Prescott, S. R. (2006). *Exploring the influence of contextual factors on the racial and ethnic identities of multiracial Asian Americans with white/European American heritage: A qualitative study.* Unpublished doctoral dissertation, Northeastern University.

Root, M. (1990). Resolving "other" status: Identity development in biracial individuals. In L. Brown & M. Root, *Diversity and complexity in feminist therapy* (pp. 185–206). Binghamton, NY: Harrington Park Press.

Root, M. (1992). Reconstructing the impact of trauma on personality. In L. Brown & M. Ballou (Eds.), *Personality and psychopathology: Feminist reappraisals* (pp. 229–266). New York: Guilford Press.

Rosewater, L., & Walker, L. (1985). *The handbook of feminist therapy.* New York: Springer Publishing.

Sellers, R., Smith, M., Shelton, J., Rowley, S., & Chavous, T. (1998). Multidimensional model of racial identity: A reconceptualization of African American racial identity. *Journal of Personality and Social Psychology Review, 2*(1), 18–39.

Sue, D. W., & Sue, D. (2003). *Counseling the culturally different: Theory and practice* (4th ed.). New York: Wiley.

Travis, C. (1992). *The mismeasure of women.* New York: Simon & Schuster.

CHAPTER 4

The Person of the Client: *Application*

Mary Ni

OVERVIEW

Barrett and Ballou, in the preceding chapter, speak about the elements and aspects of a person's life and relationships that seem so obvious when they are named. When these elements are named, help givers and help seekers can more easily see how a particular problem is related to a larger whole; they can more easily deal with a problem using multiple perspectives versus one dominant perspective. Multiple perspectives are more possible because we have a broader context from which to view the issues.

In the contextual ecological feminist model, the care-seeking individual is viewed from a wider perspective than she might be if she entered more traditional psychotherapy. A care-seeking individual is viewed from the context of how she makes sense of herself and her lived experiences in the world. Information about her understanding of herself and her life experiences is sought, as well as information about her understanding of her personal development and close relationships. Transcending the limits of traditional psychotherapy, a care-seeker is considered not only from the perspective of her relationships in her family and community systems, but also from the perspective of her relationships with broader institutions, global networks, geopolitical processes, and the physical environment.

In the context of the integrated model suggested by Barrett and Ballou, we see that rather than deal with an individual and her problems through one particular theoretical framework, we can instead use multiple models to make sense of a person's life. Through the broader lens that these models provide, we can acquire and assess a wider range of information that an individual brings to a session. Also in this context, we understand the importance of caregivers' ability to see themselves in the situation of those they are trying to help. Both caregivers and care-seekers need to be aware of themselves in the context of time, place, and circumstances. As Carol Gilligan implores us to ask, "In whose body? In what place? At what point in time?" (C. Gilligan, personal communication, January 19, 2007).

Ballou and Barrett's paradigm is used in the following three case studies, to illustrate how these questions and their implications might inform and ultimately help caregivers and care-seekers attain the relief, assistance, and other desired goals that they seek. A more fully developed focus is given to the case study of Abby. Secondary focus, to illustrate how other issues might be assisted through use of the model, is given to the case studies of Scott and of Anna and Sergei.

ABBY

In the case study of Abby, we see a young, black woman with a number of worries and problems. Her situation has raised her level of anxiety to the point that her primary care physician felt she needed antianxiety medication, which she has continued to take to the present. However, despite this medication, Abby continues to have anxiety and worries that affect her quality of life. Abby does not feel safe in her world. She worries about intruders entering her home. She worries about her mother's response to her stepfather's cancer. She worries about not being in a relationship and losing her chance to have children. She comes to therapy worried, anxious, and hoping for help.

Think Contextually

Barrett and Ballou's integrated model suggests that we consider the many angles and multiple factors of Abby's life when trying to assess and be helpful to her. Their suggestion to think contextually and act personally reminds us that we must try to see Abby and all that she is in the broadest sense. And we must also connect with her personally and well, one-on-one, in the universal, human sense.

As has been found in outcome studies of the effectiveness of psychotherapy, a most important curative factor is the relationship the client and counselor have with each other (Luborsky et al., 1971; Luborsky & Horvath, 1993). To make a good connection, we have to be able to show Abby that we are interested in her and that we care about what she has to say. We have to let her know that we are open to learning about her world and who she is. We need ultimately to care about her and convey that we do. We need to be observant of her nonverbal as well as verbal behaviors. And it would be helpful to notice not only what she says, but also the meaning in what she doesn't say. We have to be able to give her hope that her life can be better than it currently is. And we have to be able to ask good questions.

We have to be able to ask the kind of questions that show her not only that we are listening to her, but also that we are able to push her to see things from different angles and in the kinds of different ways that can help her find more effective modes of thinking and acting. In this way, using Barrett and Ballou's model, we can then begin to think, with her, of possible ways to help her reclaim her ability to move more effectively in her world.

Abby's Tapestry

From the brief description of her case, we know Abby is a complicated person. We know she is black and has two brothers, a mother, and a stepfather with colon cancer. This stepfather molested her when she was young. She had a drinking problem in college that she overcame, but she is presently on anti-anxiety drugs that seem to be a substitute for the pleasant or numbing effect that alcohol gave her. And although she has not been in a serious relationship for many years, it is inferred that Abby would like to be in a primary relationship and to also have children.

Using Barrett and Ballou's model as it relates to an individual's core identity, we want to consider how Abby embodies and identifies herself to herself. How, for instance, does she see herself (e.g., effective/ineffective, beautiful/plain, smart/stupid, strong/weak, pure/sinful, resilient/brittle, heterosexual/gay)? How does she express herself (verbally, nonverbally, and emotionally)? How would she describe herself to herself? The answers to these types of questions would give us (and perhaps also her) a better sense of how she views her own physicality, emotionality, and spirituality. Abby does describe herself as being, in part, anxious and fearful. She uses drugs, rather unsuccessfully, to try to maintain her sense of well-being. She has also begun to see a therapist in an attempt to reclaim the direction and control of her life that she seems to have lost. Her answers to the previously posed questions and her manner of answering them would help us begin to see from what point she is "stuck" in her ability to attain her goals and where we can start assisting her.

Using the next layer of the feminist ecological model (the microsystem) to organize our thoughts, we would ask Abby about her immediate environment and her day-to-day interactions with other people, including questions about her relationships with her mother, stepfather, father, and siblings. We would also inquire about her relationships with friends and neighbors, coworkers and bosses, and finally, other acquaintances and strangers with whom she interacts during the course of her daily life. The types of interactions and relationships that Abby has and has had with these people are central to her development. How has she learned to speak or not speak? What kinds of interactions are acceptable to her? As a female child of black heritage and middle-class background, what rules did she learn that she felt she needed to follow in relationship to the adults and other authority figures in her life? Given her complex relationship with her stepfather, what were the messages that she received about how she needed to be in the presence of males? And in general, how was she taught to stand up for herself?

Abby, we know, consciously remembers that she was molested three times by her stepfather. She was disturbed by his behavior but never discussed it with him or possibly anyone else, including her mother. What made her feel that she could not bring up these disturbing events to someone who could help her understand or deal with them? What lessons did these experiences teach her? That men could not be trusted? That her mother could not protect her? That she was unworthy of protection? Other things?

As Barrett and Ballou (Chapter 3 of this volume) note, "A critical component of this [microsystem] level is the recognition that a person's values and worldview are strongly influenced by the social and political views to which the person is exposed. Exploration and questioning of these influences is imperative." With this perspective in mind, some other questions related to Abby's family situation (and Barrett's second circle of identity) might be the following: What kinds of rules and traditions did she grow up with? How was she, as a girl, treated by the adults in her life? What was okay and not okay to talk about in her family? How did or does her family show affection, anger, and other strong feelings? How did she learn to treat outsiders, and how was she treated by them? How did she learn to communicate with people about things that matter? What roles did race, class, and gender play in how she learned to interact? Answers to these types of questions will help clarify Abby's sense of herself in relationship to other people. They could also clarify Abby's frame of social reference and how she views herself as a social and sexual being.

The third circle of exosystem—group identity—focuses on how more formal organizations and social policy come to affect an individual and her situations. In Abby's case, we would look at how her formal education and religious training might impact her difficulties in the present time. For example, let's hypothesize that Abby went to a conventional, small-town public school and attended a traditional Christian black church. In this scenario, Abby probably had many years of conditioning to be obedient, follow directions, and not rock the boat. She probably also experienced subtle, as well as overt, racism in her school experiences. Moreover, she probably did not learn very much about how social institutions and government can be oppressive, particularly to the working class, to people of color, to young people, and to females. Although Abby would have encountered racism and sexism, she might not have had forums in which to discuss how her experiences are related to a larger system of oppression or how they might influence and be related to her present anxieties and relational problems. Racism in the form of subtle putdowns and objectification could easily have diminished her self-esteem over time. If this is the case, it would be very helpful for Abby to become educated about the reality of systematic, institutionalized racism, sexism, and classism. She, as often happens to oppressed people, could have easily internalized oppressive concepts and started believing that the demeaning ideas, statements, and behavior toward her were true and acceptable. Given this scenario, if Abby developed a clearer understanding of how an oppressive society helped condition her into a state of helplessness and victimization, she would have the beginnings of an understanding of how to work her way free of the conditioning.

Another level of influence in the feminist contextual ecological model is the macrosystem, or global, level. The macrosystem level concerns how the relationships we develop with each other interrelate with the larger social and economic systems we experience (such as capitalism, nationalism, terrorism, multiculturalism, racism, and classism) not just locally, but worldwide. For Abby, an understanding of these interrelationships would be helpful in giving her a broader understanding of her own problems from a wider context. At the macrosystem level, as well as at the exosystem level, of understanding, Abby's heightened awareness could motivate her to connect with other people with similar difficulties. This would help her feel less alone and isolated in her situation. Moreover, it could give her reason and incentive to mobilize and empower herself to take tangible action to change the dynamics that perpetuate oppressive policies and social practices. Doing this, even in small ways, could help Abby reclaim her voice, as well as her ability to better advocate for herself and others with similar problems.

Environmental influences in the feminist contextual ecological model include how planetary conditions and the historical period in which Abby lives might affect her circumstances. Although it might seem less obvious to tie planetary conditions to Abby's anxiety, one could presuppose that the destruction and loss of life from recent natural disasters such as the tsunamis in Asia and Hurricane Katrina in the United States could contribute to Abby's anxiety and fears. Also, the historical significance of Abby's place in time could seriously affect her mood and sense of stability and control. Our current depressed economy, the Iraqi and Afghanistan wars we are waging, and violent crime all could contribute to any otherwise sane person's sense of anxiety. Many of these issues are evidence of the hegemonic, powerful structures that drive social, economic, and political policy. Fear is also a means of control and continues to be widely used as a strategy to maintain the status quo as well as to restrict civil liberties. In Abby's situation, these events could understandably contribute to a sense of job insecurity as well as general, free-floating unease.

Moreover, Abby lives in a time when she can easily obtain appropriate antianxiety medication to help her modulate her anxiety. Although this option might be useful to her, it speaks to the present-day forces of capitalism, which are linked to medical funding and research and our culturally accepted use of this type of pharmaceutical solution to psychological problems. In times past, drugs would not have been as readily available to Abby. Nor would have Western, individual psychotherapy. In times past, Abby, a young black woman, would be unlikely to have had the means or inclination to go for psychotherapy. Rather, she would have depended entirely on a combination of friends, family, pastor, herbs, and prayers. Or considering an unreceptive, unsupportive family or background, Abby may have felt she had no options at all except to suffer in silence, repress her pain, or somehow distract herself with hard work, alcohol use, or prescription or street drugs.

Finally, using the contextual ecological feminist model, I am encouraged to look at Abby through the coordinates of age, sex and gender, social and economic class, and race and ethnicity. In Abby's case, these coordinates are of a young black female from a middle-class background. Although the fact that she is able-bodied and heterosexual places her in a position of strength, her gender, youth, and blackness make her more vulnerable and more susceptible to the lack of advantages that she might otherwise enjoy were she white, middle class, and male. These latter coordinates put Abby in a position that is still less valued and more often disrespected and demeaned. They are also significant points to consider when assessing all the variables that affect Abby's well-being.

Act Personally

In using the broad perspectives of the Barrett and Ballou model to understand Abby, we can add our own experiences and training as who we are and what we bring to her situation. For example, as an experienced, yet still evolving counselor of color, this author would initially use her non-whiteness to help connect with Abby on a personal level. If Abby has assimilated white, the ethnicity of her counselor might not make much of a difference to her. But especially at first, a common understanding regarding being a minority in a majority culture could be helpful. If Abby was not assimilated white, having an aware counselor who she knew had experienced similar racial biases could be a great asset.

Educating Abby on the contextual ecological feminist model would help her frame her difficulties in a larger context. This heightened awareness of her place in the larger scheme of things could help diffuse the isolation and alienation Abby is probably feeling. Her knowledge that her anxieties and struggles are shared by many others at possibly many different levels could be both comforting and energizing and, ultimately, empowering.

When Abby theoretically understands that she is not alone in experiencing her particular types of fears and anxieties, she can then begin to build the kinds of individual and group associations that she could use to diffuse and heal from, for example, the negative effects of her molestation experiences. As we know, sexual abuse and sexual problems are often so humiliating and private that secrecy is common. To open the possibilities of discussing this and other difficult topics with caring witnesses is to begin to move to resolve the problems associated with them. Both group and individual contexts would be helpful in assisting Abby to move from unuseful, negative ways of thought to more effective thinking patterns. Similarly, Abby could be assisted to move from unuseful, negative action patterns to patterns of behaving, responding, and initiating in more proactive and empowered ways.

SCOTT

Scott, our second case study, is a 9-year-old, tall, overweight, Caucasian boy. He is a helpful, affectionate child at home but is experiencing problems at school because he doesn't like boys. He prefers girls as friends and prefers to play traditional "girls' games" such as house and dolls. Boys tease him for his effeminate qualities, and he retaliates by tripping them or otherwise seeking revenge. When his school complained about his behavior toward the other boys, Scott was referred to therapy.

How the Model Can Help Illuminate Scott's Situation

Scott, in the not-too-distant past, might have been labeled as an emotionally disturbed, gender-confused boy. Fortunately, he was born into a more accepting (yet still dangerous and demeaning) time and environment to caring, religious parents who "are tolerant of who he is." However, Scott still appears to be the major focus of negative attention and the need for discipline in his school. Despite finding himself in a situation that involves a group of aggressive boys, when Scott is taunted and teased for his feminine way of behaving, and he then retaliates, he is the one who gets in trouble, not those who were harassing him in the first place.

Using the contextual feminist ecological model to try to make sense of Scott's identity and situation, we can begin to expose the variety of forces and concerns at play in his life. These forces not only look at who Scott is as an individual, but also look more widely at the social context in which he lives. After reviewing his situation, and scanning through the layers and various elements of our model, a first question we might ask is this: does Scott really need therapy?

This question is posed when thinking about Scott's own sense of himself. To this author, Scott's response (retaliation against people who do mean things to him) seems healthy (however socially unacceptable). He doesn't take harassment silently or with a sense of resignation. It seems like Scott has a strong and positive sense of himself. He knows that his parents value him and that he is a person worthy of respect. Centered with this knowledge, he does not tolerate abuse like a doormat. Perhaps he could use some practice and techniques in more socially acceptable ways of standing up for himself, but this is different than needing therapy.

From the relational perspective, we might be concerned that the school's complaint did not address the larger dynamic of why Scott was acting out. Perhaps the school has a higher tolerance for teasing, name-calling, and other verbal assaults than it does for physical assaults. If so, this odd dichotomy needs to be looked at not only from Barrett and Ballou's relational perspectives, but also from a historical and social perspective. Name-calling and bullying behavior, continued over time, can result in tremendous violent explosions in people at whom it has been directed, who have seethed silently or quietly until the point of the vehement outburst. Remember, for example, the Columbine High School massacre of April 1999. In this troubling incident, two teenagers, Eric Harris and Dylan Klebold, plotted and executed a bloody shooting rampage in their school. In the aftermath, they both committed suicide, but not before killing 12 students and a teacher, as well as wounding 24 others. Apparently these two angry and disturbed boys had been constantly bullied and harassed, and finally, had had enough. In Scott's situation, perhaps the school administrators need mediation training so that they can deal with and resolve student conflicts without having to send students like Scott to psychotherapy.

In considering Scott from the macrosystem, or group identity, perspective, we see that Scott can easily be unprotected and set up as a target for bullying practice. This is still common in a majority culture that continues to value the concept that "might is right" so long as boys are "just beings boys" and stay under the radar. Because bullying incidents last an average of 32 seconds (Craig & Pepler, 2000), they can often go unnoticed by those in authority. Yet if our social systems and our government continue to support and model aggression and violence at the most public and international levels, and if our teachers, parents, and religious leaders say they do not back violence, but stand by silently or helplessly when it happens in the schoolyards, in our communities, and in our churches, then the message is loud and clear that if you can get away with it, it's okay to do it. If Scott, as a nontraditional student, is not protected from harassment but rather is punished for trying to defend himself, then the message is clear: it's okay to harass people who are different. If you are different and somehow stand out from the crowd, you are vulnerable and will not be supported or defended by those in power.

Using the Barrett and Ballou model in Scott's situation, we can see that his problem is not just *his* problem, but a group problem related to a broader social context and with the need for broader solutions. These solutions could include such actions as not scapegoating Scott for his retaliatory behavior, but rather applying a group educational intervention to the conflicts he is experiencing with his peers. And it could include educating the larger class (including him) on issues of tolerance, community building, and communication skills. Solutions like this would not punish Scott or label him as deficient or as a troublemaker, but instead would focus on larger group training that would, if successful, result in a more peaceable classroom and more compassionate, enlightened young people.

ANNA AND SERGEI

Anna and Sergei are working-class immigrants from Russia. They have two small children and came to the United States to follow a dream. However, this dream is falling apart as they contend with serious economic and social issues including, medical problems, unemployment, social isolation, and cultural dissonance. These stressors have understandably affected their relationship. Social services became involved after they raised their voices to each other. They were referred to therapy because of this incident.

When the stresses of life become intolerable, it is not uncommon for couples to take out their frustrations on each other. Therapeutic support can be used to deflect or release strong feelings, so that they are not displayed in harmful ways toward innocent parties. However, when people find themselves in political and economic situations that are not under their control, traditional therapy might be used to comfort and console, but more proactive social work would be more effective.

So, rather than delve into the couple's interpersonal dynamics and individual identities, it would be more useful to look at Anna and Sergei's issues from the larger social context of the contextual ecological feminist model. Anna and Sergei are devoted to each other and to their children. Their problems stem not from a need for therapeutic change, but rather from a need for more social support and political and economic change.

At the microsystem level of Anna and Sergei's immediate environment, we see that this young couple is missing an effective support system that can help them survive through hard times. Their parents and other relatives are still in Russia. They have few people around them who speak their language or understand their circumstances. The father and younger daughter need serious medical attention. And they are working as hard as possible, but are still having trouble paying the rent and may soon be homeless. They need social services more than they need individual or couple's therapy. If they could become linked to some social services that assist immigrants, and particularly Soviet immigrants, this could be the difference that allows them to stay in the United States. If they could become connected to other immigrants, if not Soviet immigrants, they might be able to exchange the kind of practical and emotional support they need to enhance their quality of life.

This couple's problems could also be easily looked at from the ecosystem level of more formal organizations and social policy. For example, services for immigrants and refugees are not well funded. The United States is presently focused on a "war on terror" and is funneling billions of dollars into military projects and aggression toward other nations who are seen as threats to our national security. With financial support wanting, many domestic needs languish. Anna and Sergei are not in a position to struggle for changes in policy and laws that would more favorably affect their circumstances. But others of us, who are in more advantageous positions, could advocate for them. If this family had access to free health care, and if they could more easily get a housing subsidy to carry them through this difficult time, it would greatly ease their present situation and relieve the terrible strain that they are currently experiencing. Although changes in policies and laws do not happen overnight, they are worth considering and striving for. Perhaps all counselors and therapists should have, as a part of their training, some classes and courses in political change toward this end. Feminist therapists, as an example, have a commitment to advocacy and social change.

CONCLUSION

The examples of Abby, Scott, and Anna and Sergei have been used to illustrate in simple ways how Barrett and Ballou's contextual ecological feminist model might be used to view individual problems from a broader context. This model can assist both care-seekers and caregivers to understand and work with human problems from the larger and more inclusive perspectives related to each individual's life.

In Abby's case, it's important to see her anxiety not only in the frame of her personality and character, but also from the context of her cultural background and the times in which she lives. In Scott's case, it would be useful not to pathologize his aggressive behavior toward his peers. Rather, in view of Scott's social environment, we could reframe his behavior in more positive ways and at the same time see the pathology in the setting in which he finds himself. Finally, in Anna and Sergei's situation, we can consider their larger social situation. Rather than assume that they are somehow deficient in their ability to make things work in their lives, we can consider the ways that the larger society is not adequately supporting their needs and can work to correct the situation from a social or communal, versus individual, level.

REFERENCES

Chesler, P. (1997). *Women and madness*. New York: Four Walls Eight Windows.

Craig, W., & Pepler, D. (2000). Observations of bullying in the playground and in the classroom school. *Psychology International 21*(1), 22–37.

De Beauvoir, S. (1953). *The second sex*. New York: Knopf.

Gilligan, C. (1982). *In a different voice*. Cambridge, MA: Harvard University Press.

Gilligan, C. (1991). Women's psychological development: Implications for psychotherapy. *Women and Therapy, 11*(3/4), 5–31.

Jackins, H. (1978). *The human side of human beings*. Seattle: Rational Island.

Laing, R. D. (1965). *The divided self*. New York: Penguin.

Luborsky, L., Chandler, M., Auerback, A. H., Cohen, J., & Bachrach, H. M. (1971). Factors influencing the outcome of psychotherapy: A review of the quantitative research. *Psychological Bulletin, 75*, 145–185.

Luborsky, L., & Horvath, A. (1993). The role of the therapeutic alliance in psychotherapy. *Journal of Consulting and Clinical Psychology, 61*(4), 561–573.

Miller, J. B. (1987). *Towards a new psychology of women*. Boston: Beacon Press.

CHAPTER 5

The Practice of Psychotherapy: *Theory*

Lauren Gentile, Susie Kisber, Jaime Suvak, and Carolyn West[1]

In the domain of therapy, theory is commonly understood to be a set of assumptions on which rest the practitioner's understandings about human behavior, about what constitutes mental health and illness, and about the various factors to which an individual's status may be attributed. Theory also serves to inform not only the strategies and techniques that are employed but, in more subtle ways, also the manner in which the therapist interfaces with the client; the artifacts of therapy in the way of forms and procedures, for example; and even the therapist's expectations of a client's prognosis. That is, theory informs the way in which the therapist thinks about a client and the way in which the actual therapy is conducted in the particular and in the broadest sense, as well.

The ways in which therapy is linked to its companion theory and the contrast between traditional therapies and feminist therapy are reminiscent of what is termed a contemporary fable, and a fable is here adapted for this current discussion.

---

1. This chapter was a collaborative work. The authors are listed in alphabetical order.

UPSTREAM/DOWNSTREAM

It was many years ago that the villagers of Downstream spotted the first body in the river. Some old-timers remember how limited the techniques and resources were for managing that sort of thing. Sometimes, they recall, it would take hours to pull 10 people from the river, and even then only a few would survive.

Though the number of victims in the river has increased dramatically over the years, the good folks of Downstream are responding admirably to the challenge. Their rescue system and the industries that support them flourish. Many people discovered in the swirling waters are reached within 20 minutes—and some in less than 10. Each day fewer are drowning before help arrives—a big improvement from the way it used to be.

Talk to the people of Downstream, and they'll speak with pride about the modern complex by the edge of the waters, the flotilla of rescue boats ready for service at a moment's notice, the large numbers of highly trained swimmers at the ready to save victims, and, in recent years, the ubiquity of little pills, promising refuge from the effects of the raging currents.

Oh, a few people in Downstream have raised the question now and again, but most folks show little interest in what's happening Upstream. It seems there's so much to do just to tend Downstream to help those in the river that nobody's got time to check into how all those bodies are getting in there in the first place. That's just the way things are.

As the fable reminds us, in many ways, where we look—or conversely, where we fail to look—determines what we find, what we choose to do, and also what remains unseen and therefore unconsidered. Theoretical orientations preceding the advent of feminist therapy in the 1970s focused on the individual and, to some very limited extent, the individual's context and system membership as it related primarily to family. Regardless of the explanations of mainstream or "Downstream" theories regarding the origins or causes of mental illness, a common denominator has been the unexamined acceptance of the ways in which the larger culture operates, an at best naive collusion with the status quo, a failure to deconstruct the invisible cultural and sociopolitical assumptions that determine who gets how much of what—education, employment, housing, and health care, for example—as well as the less measurable but critically influential commodities of opportunity, power, protection, and, not unimportantly, regard. Theories that stop short of this critical analysis spawn interventions that can have only a limited impact, akin to the people of Downstream who build new boats or invent new rescue techniques or who decide, in the moment of crisis, who gets saved.

It has been said elsewhere that in practice feminist therapy draws from a wide range of possible interventions, many familiar to or consistent with other theoretical models. As demonstrated by Barrett and Ballou (Chapter 3 of this volume), feminist therapy attends to the individual and to the near levels of context—the family, the community, the school, and so on—*and* feminist therapy uniquely and conscientiously and by its very definition situates the client with careful, thoughtful, searching attention to sociopolitical, economic, and cultural forces. To continue the analogy, feminist therapy may have a flotilla Downstream, but its primary operation and its impassioned efforts are Upstream.

Feminist therapy theory insists on this broader analysis, not only looking at context, but also challenging the very operating system of that context—its assumptions and beliefs, its hierarchical arrangements and inequities, and its links to power and privilege and the oppressions that form and metastasize in their shadows. The framework that informs the work of feminist therapy is constructed of a set of principles that provide the therapist with not only a way of thinking about a client but also a way of applying or offering a wide array of interventions. From a feminist therapy perspective, it is less about whether a particular intervention is "feminist" and more about the thinking that is used in selecting and implementing the intervention.

These principles, rooted in sociopolitical tenets (Ballou & West, 2000; Hill & Ballou, 1998), and the ways in which they guide and shape feminist therapy practice form the basis for the theory of feminist psychotherapy and are the subject of this chapter. It is noted that the principles and the intentions they foster are not discrete entities, nor are they hard and fast rules or injunctions; rather they are an overlapping and complementary set of guidelines, together offering a way of doing the work of therapy, with care and often imperfectly, which is aimed consistently in the direction of fairness and equity and justice.

THE VALUING OF ALL EXPERIENCE

Feminist therapy is unwaveringly rooted in the search for and valuing of the experiences of *all* people (Ballou & West, 2000; Hill & Ballou, 1998). With an awareness that initially emerged from their own experience as women in a patriarchal culture, feminist therapists recognize that the experiences of majority cultures have long been viewed as the norm and often as the only valid perspective. Women's voices and the experiences of nonwhites have historically been overlooked by dominant, purportedly apolitical psychotherapy theories, and the premises of these theories were and are used as the platform for working with—or perhaps a more precise preposition would be "on"—these marginalized groups. This practice of assumptive treatment has as its consequence a further cementing of one's marginalized status and the continued silencing of already muted voices.

With the critical awareness that forms the basis of its theory brought to bear on itself, feminist theory expanded in its early years, from its attention to white, middle-class women, to a focus that includes women of color as well. Looking back from our current vantage, some of the earlier focuses of feminist therapy seem quite obvious, and attention to them now is more mainstream. Considering the continuum of violence, for example, topics such as domestic violence and sexual harassment have entered the lexicon of institutions such as health care and the judicial system, and although the response continues to be imperfect, nonetheless, some degree of awareness is penetrating the culture.

In today's increasingly globalized society, however, the critical analysis that is feminist theory's hallmark continues to challenge unexamined assumptions and injustice based on this first principle of the valuing of all experience. And the analysis has become increasingly complex as theory builders consider multiple layers of identity and experience. Importantly, feminist theory has remained fluid and malleable, broadening and deepening to include other voices as they have been listened for and have made themselves heard. This is an ongoing, sometimes raucous, always enlightening, and frequently humbling process. It involves awareness, discussion, reflection, openness, and willingness. It is seldom tidy, often painful, and never complete.

In a culture that prizes knowledge and status, this principle of the valuing of all experience encourages practitioners to be aware of their own culturally inculcated and faulty assumptions without believing or acting on them, to value the person with whom they are sitting as the expert on her or his own experience, and to listen and consider respectfully and from a place of not-knowing—looking for ways to connect across the "space between" (Josselson, 1995, p. 6). This not-knowing includes the further identification of culturally bound assumptions about what is considered best for this person, when often what is considered best from a Downstream perspective—that which is unstated, yet politically shaped—is that the client conform more fully with the sociopolitical landscape, as is. Metaphorically, she or he is welcomed *in* the rescue boat, but is certainly not allowed to rock it! In the practice of feminist therapy, however, the understanding of what actions and changes are called for and how these are to be implemented are allowed to arise from the collaborative joining with the client.

This collaboration includes a transparency about the process of therapy itself. Feminist therapists often explicitly state their values, in print or in conversation, engage in explanations about their thinking, and check in with their clients about their experiences, thoughts, and feelings. In contrast to the image of the knowing expert, the relationship does not revolve around "treating" or "doing to"; rather it is a joint, negotiated effort intended to arrive at a client-oriented definition of what "better" feels like and what changes need to occur in order to access this. The aims of this exchange are honesty, clarity, and collaboration.

VALUING INDIVIDUAL DIFFERENCES

Although continuing to shine the light of a thorough and critical analysis on issues of gender, the evolution of feminist therapy has been characterized by a broadening of awareness to include additional categories of oppression as well as a refinement of attention that examines the ways in which membership in multiple categories influences one's experience. This pulsation between naming the universal categories of oppression—for example, the poor, people of color, the infirm, or the elderly—and noting the uniqueness of a particular constellation of multiple identities encompassing, perhaps, all of these categories, represents feminist therapy's commitment to each within the context of all.

In sum, there is an appreciation in feminist therapy for the uniqueness *as well as* the commonality of each person's story, and a goal of the therapeutic relationship is to engage with clients in a holistic way that acknowledges and respects the multiple aspects of their experience. Barrett and Ballou in Chapter 3 of this volume set out a useful model for conceptualizing multiple layers of influence and identity, a way of considering the individual within context(s) that contrasts with more linear, narrowly framed, more static developmental models.

While acknowledging that there is undoubtedly more work to be done, and more layers to be attended to, this current conceptualization is considerably broader, more thorough, and more textured than that of feminist theory's origins—the naming and treatment of oppression experienced by (white, mostly middle-class) women and girls; yet what remains central and continues to inform all thinking is that mental health, the quality of life, and one's general well-being are influenced and compromised by living in a culture based on sexism, misogyny, and uneven access to power and privilege (Ballou & Brown, 2002; Brown, 1994; Brown & Ballou, 1992; Hill & Ballou, 2005; Jordan, Hartling, & Walker, 2004; Kaschak, 1992; Miller, 1976; Miller, Walker, & Rosen, 2004).

One example of an area involving individual difference in which feminist psychotherapy theory has broadened over time follows a shift from the conceptualization of gender as binary to the consideration and recognition of a wide continuum of gender expression (Bornstein, 1998; Fausto-Sterling, 2000; Feinberg, 1999; Kessler, 1998). As more people, bravely, perhaps, live in ways that express their own uniqueness and that challenge mainstream ideas and theoretical models of gender and sexuality, feminist therapists are noting and naming what appears to be a rise in gender-based hate crimes and violence and the prevalence of religiously cloaked political forces mobilized under the guise of the "protection of family values."

And here, too, can be seen both the struggle inherent in revising, adjusting, and expanding theory and the richness of more fully elaborated thought and understanding. For example, an increased number of people identifying as transgender and the emergence of a large female-to-male (FTM) community, including FTMs who previously identified as lesbians, has challenged feminist theory to deconstruct the definitions of male and female, examining and exploring previously held assumptions and the biases they disguised (Bornstein, 1998; Fausto-Sterling, 2000; Feinberg, 1999). In early feminism, male-to-female (MTF) transsexuals were often responded to as colonizers of women and were not welcome in the feminist and women's community. Likewise, FTMs were seen by many as women betraying their sisters in order to assume masculine privilege. Current feminist therapy theory is working toward becoming more sensitive to and embracing the complexities that transgender identities present.

This represents one example of continuing shifts and new developments in gender that are providing opportunities to widen the lens of feminist therapy theory, understand "interlocking vectors" of diversity and oppressions, and deepen the understanding of gender and sexuality (personal communication, Hill, January 12, 2007). A sampling of other areas where feminist theory is expanding and developing includes work with incarcerated women (Leeder, 2006), classism (Hill & Rothblum, 1996), biracial issues (Gillem & Thompson, 2004), and black women and violence (West, 2002).

REDRESSING POWER DIFFERENTIALS

If theory were to be distilled to a single word or concept, then in regard to feminist theory, "power" would offer itself as a likely candidate. Abuses of power, power over, and disempowerment are all variations of the concept that feminist theory recognizes as a critical Upstream phenomenon. Power is wielded both knowingly and unknowingly by those who have it, to keep their goods, their status, their influence, the primacy of their ideology and culture, and—in the current political climate—the illusion of their safety. The theory of feminist psychotherapy has historically identified and continues to accommodate to the many ways in which power over does harm, separating and defining and stratifying; on an individual level, feminist therapy seeks to provide an experience of shared power or power "with."

The theme of power over and its destructive force is illuminated in various ways throughout each of the feminist therapy principles. Feminist therapy theory posits that the imbalance of power and privilege inherent in society is core to psychological distress (Ballou & Brown, 2002; Brown, 1994; Jordan et al., 2004; Kaschak, 1992; Miller, 1976; Miller, Walker, & Rosen, 2004). Since its inception, feminist therapy has evolved in order to meet the needs of clients in a society whose structural and oppressive forces continue to impact the well-being of individuals. The purported objectivity of Downstream therapies and their companion science is maintained and perpetuated by the failure of such thinking to critique the culture that supports it. On the other hand, feminist theory acknowledges that therapy is a value-laden process, and feminist therapists do their best to explicate their own context and values. A core value is to maintain an integrated analysis of the impact that oppression and access to power and privilege has on people's lives (Hill & Ballou, 1998).

Feminist theory demands a critical analysis at the macro level regarding the socioeconomic, cultural, and political forces that impact a particular client, as well as at the micro level of the therapeutic relationship and experience. Hart, in this volume, provides an in-depth exploration of both established procedures and moment-to-moment considerations within the encounter between therapist and client that provide opportunities not only to avoid the perpetuation of power-over injuries, but also to empower within the relationship itself by encouraging client authority and assertiveness.

This overarching attention to power is easily stated but complicated in practice, demanding of the therapist a continual critical awareness. As pointed out by Roffman in this volume, the current reality, itself a reflection of the dominant social paradigm, is that white, middle-class therapists are largely those responsible for providing services to clients who may be different in terms of social, economic, and political power. Noting this imbalance, feminist theory dictates the therapist's responsibility to seek consultation, education, and training to address the blind spots arising from her own history and experiences and to sift through the tiers of vulnerability (Hart, 2006) that present within her and within the therapeutic encounter. This is not only a central tenet of feminist theory, but a core ethical issue as well.

CONTEXTUALIZING THE CAUSES OF
EMOTIONAL DISTRESS

"Feminist therapy recognizes a primary need to consider behaviors and intra-psychic processes as they are embedded within a sociopolitical context" (Ballou & West, 2000, p. 274). Importantly, the Feminist Therapy Institute's Code of Ethics (1990, 1999) was the first of its kind to communicate that it is a therapist's ethical responsibility to attend to the sociopolitical context of people's lives.

"Context" is a term that has certainly made its way Downstream, and it would indeed be a rare therapist of any theoretical orientation who would not consider a client's context to be relevant. But terms and their applications over time can become neutralized, their precision blunted, their impact diluted such that the commonly agreed-upon meaning fits more neatly into the dominant culture's lexicon. So Downstream, the consideration of context may involve noting the circles of influence—for example, family relationships, community ties, employment, and financial status—that impact the client's presenting problems; and subsequently, the client can be helped to modify her responses, to fit more acceptably, to adopt a repertoire of coping strategies, and even to adjust her biochemistry such that symptoms are reduced. What is *not* considered, however, is that context in this regard itself bears examination. That context itself is part of the problem: there is a context to the context.

Feminist theory acknowledges a major distinction between taking note of the context of behavior—for example, noting that Scott's gender-different behaviors are the target of teasing—and situating this youngster within the broad context of a culture where the expectations for gendered behavior are binary and rigid. Context is both narrow and immediate (in this case, the context of a classroom and community) and broader and more universal (in this case, harmful and biased sociocultural structures that insidiously inform Scott's self-view and the expectations and reactions of others to him). Feminist theory contextualizes by both seeing through and seeing into.

At the level of practice, feminist therapists often inquire about the meaning that context has for those involved. Many times, the therapist's role is to help people hold different versions of how they understand contextual variables and to sit with this ambiguity. There is an inherent valuing and supporting of the pursuit of authenticity over the adherence to socially proscribed norms. For example, a feminist therapist is likely to challenge a person's culturally inculcated belief that depression is completely biologi-cal and instead encourage consideration of the impact the person's daily experiences and relationships have on her or his mood. The therapist might encourage someone to take her or his feelings of being trapped or unappreciated seriously as factors underlying that person's depression. This is but one example of how feminist therapists continually work to take into account interlocking multiple layers of experience and the complexities of relationships. Their attention to context takes note of the particular circumstances of an individual's distress, while simultaneously deconstructing its sociopolitical operating system.

QUESTIONING NORMS AND STANDARDS OF MENTAL HEALTH

Because the research and standards that govern traditional models of mental health, including its definitions, its practices, its treatment protocols, and even its theoretical underpinnings, are embedded within the social system it presumes to help, the discipline itself serves to affirm and maintain the status quo. Operating Downstream, traditional models treat casualties of the sociopolitical structures in a way that often best serves the needs of the culture rather than the individual. Treatment for Scott, for example, may yield the adoption of behaviors more typical of a masculine stereotype and may result in a less disruptive classroom. The unseen and unacknowledged cost, however, would be the devaluing of individual difference and the short- and long-term consequences of that to Scott, as well as the reinforcement of gender stereotypes and the perpetuation, indeed the affirmation, of a system of marginalization and abuse.

Throughout the history of psychology, and intensifying in the political climate of the last decade, has been a reduction of human experience to that which can be identified and measured by the golden calf of objective science. Experience and behavior that differ from norms as established by the powerful are viewed as deviant or disordered or are not viewed at all. Indeed, this type of research often renders invisible the many intersecting variables operating in people's lives. Mirroring this narrowing of what defines health is the current language of mental health treatment concerned with validated studies, outcome measures, and standardized protocols.

As discussed earlier, feminist therapy theory values personal experience and the consciousness that develops as a result of this experience, and it is routinely and necessarily skeptical of traditionally held "objective truths." Normative data gathered by a scientific community that considers itself objective and value-free offer only what can be grossly considered typical among those who were studied rather than providing reliable indicators of healthy, correct, or desired behavior (Ballou & Brown, 2002). Just as the establishment of an average occludes the continuum from which the average was derived, this unnamed and unexamined value-laden system of categorization exerts unrealistic expectations on those in the majority and marginalizes those who live their lives apart from the mainstream culture.

Traditional methodologies also sacrifice the individual to the membership of the group, thus obscuring the individual differences that feminist theory considers essential. Indeed, feminist theory is cautious regarding all aspects of the scientific illusion—of empirically validated answers to universal questions as investigated by neutral observers (Ballou & Brown, 2002)—because even the research questions that are framed say something about the values of the researcher, about the social biases of the sponsors of the research, and ultimately about who and what is important. Stakeholders who are funding or promoting research agendas are rarely forthcoming about their interests and biases, and researchers who may themselves have membership in institutions wielding power and its sidekick, privilege, are potentially influenced by several layers of bias, including the personal, the institutional, and the political. Under such conditions, truth and authenticity are remote or only partial visitors. With its focus on experience, a feminist perspective considers qualitative and mixed research designs that locate the researcher within the sociopolitical landscape, clear a space for the voice of the participant, and, in optimal situations, provide some benefit to the individual as well as to a more complete understanding of the social order in which she lives.

Not surprisingly, traditional, empirically grounded science yields interventions that contain the same individual and social assumptions and biases; feminist theory naturally regards these, too, with caution. Outcome measures, which can be akin to keeping records regarding the number of Downstream rescues, are increasingly important in the domain of mental health, and the emphasis here can result in service providers and clients not being valued for the important work being done in non-empirically oriented treatments. Efficiency, translated as short-term or brief therapy, and measurable efficacy, translated as, for example, reduced recidivism and employee absence, are themes that drive not only the awarding of research grants but the policies of most health insurance companies as well. Feminist therapy, on the other hand, relies more on a conjoint, less institutionally driven assessment of progress in therapy. Consistent with feminist therapy's regard for process and shared power, a feminist discernment would involve discussion of what has been considered, felt, and understood by the most critically important people—those in the relationship.

To some extent these differences between mainstream and feminist therapies in the manner in which outcomes are determined has to do with very basic perspectives on what constitutes health and wellness. For example, feminist therapists strive to understand what meaning the reduction of the symptoms of posttraumatic stress disorder may have for a client in a society that remains potentially dangerous. Although a traditional outcome measure may see symptom reduction as a measure of success—the person has been hauled into the rescue boat—feminist therapy would look beyond symptomatology by attending to such things as what the client may be giving up to become "healthy" and to an exploration and understanding of the structural elements of society that have contributed to the client's distress.

Because of its commitment to the deconstruction of sociopolitical forces and its recognition of the many faces of harm resulting from increasing levels of power over, many feminists feel that the idea of "treatment" in regard to the individual is in and of itself disempowering because it can deny a person's agency and confine the locus of the problem to the individual. Indeed, a fabled version of feminist therapy might see the more appropriate client as the culture, with outcomes being measured in terms of shared power and universal respect. Still, many feminist therapists note that clients feel legitimized, liberated, and less stigmatized as they increasingly see their concerns as "treatable." Others report that therapy has brought them an increased sense of empowerment because they have been partners in treatment to improve their lives.

This should not be interpreted as a complete rejection of empirical research and treatments. Rather, feminist theory, with its emphasis on context, naturally attends to the context of research as well, noting that the "truth" of empirically derived data as it is framed by scientific legitimacy is also part of a larger context. Feminist theory recognizes that complex concerns can easily be sacrificed to conditions of experimental control (Ballou & Brown, 2002), and the reliance on research that is neither multifaceted nor client-centered risks the decontextualization of people's lives and an unwitting collusion with the relevant sociocultural and political realities.

THE IMPERATIVE OF SOCIAL CHANGE

Social justice and activism are core values of feminist theory. Feminist therapists explicitly acknowledge that the personal is political and that conversely the political is personal (Brown & Ballou, 1992). In other words, what one experiences personally is part of a larger political tapestry, and what happens on the political and social landscape impacts the individual's psyche and behavior in ways often neither seen nor acknowledged. As repeated throughout this text, feminist therapists form an intention and direct efforts toward the central value of human rights, seeking to change the existing power structure and hierarchical nature of society. These efforts challenge all forms of oppression in an effort to dismantle the power-over society and transform it into a power-sharing culture (Miller & Stiver, 1998), working toward both an end to oppression at the individual and systemic levels and the achievement of equality and peace.

Each and every interaction then, as viewed through a feminist lens, has political meaning, and the practices that flow out of this perspective—the sharing of the analysis of power and the questioning of the status quo—are radical when compared with traditional therapies. At an individual level such a practice is infused by an intention to effect, in the words of Susan Barrett (2006), "radical change in a liberal manner over time." Although this often has affected one therapist and one client at a time, the scope is more apparent when considering, for example, such writings as the anthology of feminist therapy theorists that defines, in various voices, therapy as a political act (Hill, 1998).

Additionally, feminist theory extends the ethical responsibility of the therapist outward, beyond the office, bringing an analysis of power to such seemingly mainstream endeavors as consultation as well as to teaching, testing, and research. These, too, are regarded as politically imbued from a feminist perspective, and engagement in these processes carries with it both the opportunity and the responsibility to engage in political activism. There is a recognition, of course, that not all feminist therapists will engage in research or hold formal teaching positions, and there is an encouragement to express the tenet of social action and expanded practice consistent with one's style, strengths, and situation. The analyses of case examples in this handbook offer a sampling of possibilities, of activities, of ideas and efforts, and of advocacy and psychoeducation representing the diversity of therapist responses directed toward the fundamental goal of equality. From the early days of the feminist therapy movement and continuing today, social workers in particular are known for their commitment to this process.

Throughout their history, feminist therapists too have been at the forefront of the political movements aimed at strengthening legislation and increasing awareness about a variety of human rights and social justice issues. They have, for example, called attention to the prevalence and severity of sexual violence and have advocated for laws that provide protection to such vulnerable populations as children (Anderson & Hill, 1997), elders (Davis, Cole, & Rothblum, 1993), the differently abled (Olkin, 1999), and those involved in domestically abusive relationships (Walker, 2000). Feminist therapists have also pioneered research and treatment for trauma survivors (Herman, 1993) and, through efforts to curtail sexist, homophobic, and racist psychological diagnoses, have challenged the mainstream psychological community to examine the ways in which minorities have been pathologized (Ballou & Brown, 2002; Brown & Root, 1990; Brown, 1994; Comas-Diaz & Greene, 1994; Greene & Herek, 1994; Jackson & Greene, 2000; Jordan, 1997; Jordan et al., 2004; Kaschak, 1992; Miller, 1976; Miller, Walker, & Rosen, 2004).

The specific issues mobilizing attention and action are, of course, impacted by the times and world events. For example, as a result of the HIV epidemic and its treatment over the last 20 years, medical activism has become more prevalent and sophisticated. Such feminist principles as those relative to individual difference and hierarchical relationships, which guided the initial response to this crisis, are used to challenge the Downstream response to mental and physical health care.

During this first decade of the twenty-first century, there is, for example, both an expansion and a refinement of attention to women's health, addressing such concerns as the medicalization of normal developmental processes, including menstruation and perimenopause (Chrisler, 2004). And current activism in this regard can be witnessed when feminist organizations refuse state funding in order to avoid the stipulated regulatory control that would reinforce and perpetuate efforts to control women's health and individual choices. While we are writing this book, legislation limiting abortion has passed the Congress and has been signed by the president. This legislation concerns a specific kind of abortion but is part of the campaign to control women's bodies in the United States. The issues change, with gains that cannot be assumed won and that are at times co-opted by the mainstream community. Feminist therapy's attention to not only each client but also the forces that impact each client extends both out of theoretical principles and from an ethical ethos.

As a result of their efforts beyond the office, the ethical standards of feminist therapists have also influenced practice in several areas of mainstream psychology. Importantly, feminist therapists were among the first to advocate for true informed consent for mental health treatment (Lerman & Porter, 1990). Also, such work as that of Gartrell (1994) and Rave and Larsen (1995) serves to articulate the ethics and modes of practice that consider multiple interlocking layers of oppression and the complexities of relationships. It is also important to acknowledge that feminist therapy has itself been influenced by such groups as womanists, multicultural feminists, and liberation psychologists. The perspectives of these groups have been critical to the continued shaping of feminist theory, particularly when considering collaboration with disenfranchised groups such as people of color and the GLBT community. This is congruent with the values of feminist therapists to celebrate difference, advocate for human rights, and address abuse of power.

FEMINIST PRACTICE AND DOWNSTREAM APPROACHES

The principles that ground feminist theory contain in their articulation many of the ways in which feminist therapy practice is different from mainstream approaches. The following points are offered to bring further definition to these differences, to some of the similarities, and to the ways in which feminist theory has influenced mainstream practice.

Most mainstream psychological perspectives are based on linear developmental models that focus on what is considered the ultimate goal of separation and individuation. With this as a starting point, one possible objective of therapy may be to strengthen individual boundaries and to foster autonomy and separateness. In a capitalist society, this goal turns out to be eerily consonant with the notions of individual success and achievement, with the accumulation of wealth and possessions, and with the pursuit and retention of power.

In contrast, feminist therapists regard connectedness as an essential feature of being human and consider increasingly complex relationships to be the result and the goal of healthy development. From this perspective human beings thrive when connected and suffer when disconnected from themselves and others. One branch of feminist therapy, relational cultural theory (RCT), suggests that therapy itself is one such relationship and that the mutuality experienced in the therapeutic process is critically important to the healing process. Mutuality is defined here as "having an impact on the other, seeing that our actions, feelings, or thoughts affect the other and opening to the influence of others on us" (Jordan, 1991, p. 88).

This perspective influences not only how the feminist therapist thinks about a client in terms of the strength and quality of relationships, but also how the therapy itself is conducted. RCT theorists believe that it is imperative for a client to feel that the therapist is impacted by the client as well as connected to and actively engaged in the therapeutic exchange (Miller & Stiver, 1998); and a key element to connectedness and engagement is mutual empathy. Therapy then is an active process that includes providing attention and presence in the moment, listening to and acknowledging objective knowledge, and seeking to understand the experience of the individual. And within this exchange, the therapist allows the client to see that she has been moved by—has felt with—the client. The emphasis on the relational aspects of therapy is intended to offer a model of healthy connection as well as to address and work toward healing the common societal experiences of shame, humiliation, marginalization, objectification, and alienation.

This way of viewing the therapeutic relationship makes room for judicious self-disclosure about "in-the-moment" experiences with a client as a way to explore relational aspects of the therapeutic alliance or the client's distress. And feminist therapists, with an emphasis on authenticity and shared power, are open to being seen as human and fallible (Hill, 1998; Hill & Rothblum, 1996) rather than degreed and omnipotent. With this level of intimacy in the therapeutic encounter, it is important for feminist therapists to engage in consultation and to be unwavering in keeping the client's welfare as the focus of treatment (Miller, Jordan, Stiver, Walker, Surry, & Eldridge, 2004).

Feminist therapists try to reconfigure the therapeutic encounter to be collaborative in a variety of ways. Although this is no longer unique to feminist therapy, its origins lie in feminist theory. With traditional therapies and in spite of attention to the therapist–client relationship, the therapeutic relationship is often set up with the therapist in an "expert" role, teaching clients how to manage the "problems" in their lives. This hierarchical relationship leaves the client in a position of disempowerment, mirroring the power dynamics of society at large (Hill & Ballou, 1998).

As can be conjectured from the foregoing principles, the very notion of diagnosis from a feminist perspective is often quite different from mainstream approaches, and the feminist insistence on looking Upstream to understand experience is often discordant with Downstream's very real need to work with insurance companies and managed care protocols. Discussed in detail elsewhere in this volume, feminist therapy resists the routine, often mechanized and power-over categorization of experience into the rigid parameters of the *Diagnostic and Statistical Manual of Mental Disorders* (*DSM-IV*, 2000), a diagnostic manual that many regard as a dictionary of disease. Though acknowledging that developmental patterns and biological data are relevant in considering the issues people present, feminist therapists recognize the need to look at these issues in multiple ways and work with clients to analyze the impact of society on their psychological well-being.

This is distinctly different from assessing a client's problems from the perspective of a medical model or even health psychology. In these two disciplines, the "expert" therapist would assess and treat the patient. From a feminist perspective, the process of "naming" the distress of a particular client is a collaborative effort to understand how the current, standard diagnostic system would conceptualize their issues rather than participating in the detached and power-laden process of diagnosis and labeling (Ballou & West, 2000).

Mainstream therapies are often primarily symptom-focused, seeking improved functioning or effecting a better fit within the client's contextual milieu. A Downstream psychotherapeutic approach to treating depression, for example, may be to work with the client to change negative thoughts with sparse attention to their origins, or to encourage and support the practice of medicating away the feelings of depression. Although either of these tools—cognitive reframing or psychopharmacology—may also be used within a feminist model of treatment, there would be unflinching attention to the possibility that the individual symptoms of a client's depression may represent the client's personal experience of oppression. This is truly the difference between support that emanates from a thoroughly Downstream perspective and support that insists on an awareness of Upstream phenomena.

As mentioned previously, feminist therapy holds a broader view of the definition of successful therapy. For example, a rape survivor may be helped by a feminist therapist to look beyond symptom reduction to the exploration of such issues as how the larger culture contributes to the continuum of violence of which rape is a part and what it means to live in a world where women are sexually objectified and sexual assault is common. There might also be discussions about the client's anger, about what it means to her that angry women are often pathologized or demeaned, and about the widespread cultural discomfort with the overt expression of anger by women. Whether the client wants to engage in criminal proceedings and the potential for this to be re-traumatizing might also be discussed. Such conversations offer a deeper layer of meaning to the therapeutic process than a primary attention to symptom reduction.

Many feminist practices have been mainstreamed into what is commonly thought of as best practice. These practices include working collaboratively with clients, culturally contextualizing clients' concerns, making a commitment to cultural competency, fully considering a client's trauma history when assessing and diagnosing, and obtaining a thorough informed consent. When the mainstream community adopts or co-opts feminist practices and language, however, the content may be loosely retained while the essence is lost or distorted.

One example would be the use of a thorough consent form written in easily understandable language. This practice emerged out of a feminist intention to engage the client from the earliest contact in a therapeutic process that is collaborative, transparent, and respectful. Yet the translation of this practice into mainstream work is often precipitated by the desire to protect therapists if their work comes under institutional scrutiny. As well, listening to clients' stories and helping them formulate a retelling from a more empowered perspective is a technique currently attributed to the school of narrative therapy, but its roots are situated firmly in early feminist therapy (Hill & Ballou, 1998). And because many of the current versions of narrative therapy do not attend to the sociopolitical context of a problem, the original feminist essence is compromised.

Historically, the needs of the therapist have not been considered a significant part of the therapeutic exchange. Feminist therapy was one of the first in the field to consider the person of the therapist and to voice the need for therapists to participate in self-care (Feminist Therapy Institute, 1999). Self-care involves, of course, attention to one's own well-being within a field that bears an insistent, relentless witness to the casualties of injustice.

Additionally, if one believes in the importance of configuring the therapeutic relationship to be as equalitarian as possible and believes that mutuality is one of the healing elements of therapy, then the importance of the therapist's stating and honoring her own boundaries naturally follows. Judith Jordan writes about "stating [one's] limits rather than setting limits on the other person" (Miller, Jordan, et al., 2004, p. 71) as a responsible and authentic way to take care of oneself and model self-care for clients. She also points out that therapy relationships, like any other type of relationship, demand that clients attend to their own needs while also respecting the needs of others. Negotiating this in therapy can be a growth-producing experience. The therapist who honestly evaluates her limits and honors them is more able to be authentically present and available for the client over time.

In summary, the principles of feminist therapy theory provide its definition as a truly contextualized model in that the individual is situated amid the multiplicity of sociopolitical forces that impinge and impact, shape and distort, select and cull, and include and exclude; and feminist therapy serves both this client, the one who has sought or been sent for help, and those others who are oppressed in similar ways. It is consonant with traditional therapies, those operating Downstream, in its use of a particular technique or strategy, yet it employs that technique with the feminist sensibility keyed into shared power and collaboration.

Feminist therapy is fully formed and substantial, and it is fluid and expanding. It is rooted in the feminist legacy of previous generations, and it is open to and integrates emerging ideas from multicultural, critical, queer, postmodern, systems, and dialectical theories (Ballou, Matsumoto, & Wagner, 2002) as well as cognitive behavioral (Hill & Ballou, 1998) and psychobiological therapies (Worell & Remer, 2003). Originally feminist therapy was the sole discipline in the field of psychology to address the impact of uneven access to power and privilege. Now with the advent of multiculturalism and social justice, the fourth and fifth forces within the counseling field (personal communication, Singh, January 30, 2007; Ratts, D'Andrea, & Arredondo, 2004), this commitment to advocacy is widening and strengthening.

Feminist theory has long realized that what is happening Upstream matters critically. It has always known that simply treating the symptomatic sequelae of oppression not only leaves the oppressive forces intact, but also serves to reinforce them, to strengthen them. And it recognizes that as we enter the twenty-first century, the current climate of domination and conservatism requires the joining and collaborative efforts of like-minded individuals to expose and challenge the way things work—both Upstream *and* Downstream.

REFERENCES

American Psychiatric Association. (2000). *Diagnostic and statistical manual of mental Disorders* (4th ed., text rev.). Washington, DC: Author.

Anderson, G., & Hill, M. (1997). *Children's rights, therapists' responsibilities: Feminist commentaries.* Binghamton: Haworth Press.

Ballou, M., & Brown, L. (Eds.). (2002). *Rethinking mental health and disorder: Feminist perspectives.* New York: Guildford Press.

Ballou, M., Matsumoto, A., & Wagner, M. (2002). Toward a feminist ecological theory of human nature. In M. Ballou & L. Brown (Eds.), *Rethinking mental health and disorder* (pp. 99–141). New York: Guildford Press.

Ballou, M., & West, C. K. (2000). Feminist therapy approaches. In M. Biaggio & M. Hersen (Eds.), *Issues in the psychology of women.* New York: Kluwer Academic/Plenum.

Barrett, S. (2006, November). Remarks presented at the Advanced Feminist Therapy Institute, Dayton, OH.

Bornstein, K. (1998). *My gender workbook.* New York: Routledge.

Brown, L. (1994). *Subversive dialogues: Theory in feminist therapy.* New York: Basic Books.

Brown, L., & Ballou, M. (Eds.). (1992). *Personality and psychopathology: Feminist reappraisals.* New York: Guildford Press.

Brown, L., & Root, M. (Eds.). (1990). *Diversity and complexity in feminist therapy.* Binghamton: Haworth Press.

Chrisler, J. C. (2004). Introduction. *Women in Therapy, 27*(3/4), 1–3.

Cole, E., Rothblum, E., & Erdman, E. (Eds.). *Wilderness therapy for women: The power of adventure.* Binghamton: Haworth Press.

Comas-Diaz, L., & Greene, B. (Eds.). (1994). *Women of color: Integrating ethnic and gender identities in psychotherapy.* New York: Guilford Press.

Davis, N., Cole, E., & Rothblum, E. (Eds.). (1993). *Faces of women and aging.* Binghamton: Haworth Press.

Fausto-Sterling, A. (2000). *Sexing the body: Gender politics and the construction of sexuality.* New York: Basic Books.

Feinberg, L. (1999). *Trans liberation: Beyond pink or blue.* Boston: Beacon Press.

Feminist Therapy Institute. (1999). *Feminist therapy code of ethics.* Retrieved from http://www.feminist-therapy-institute.org/ethics.htm

Gartrell, N. (Ed.). (1994). *Bringing ethics alive: Feminist ethics in psychotherapy practice.* Binghamton: Haworth Press.

Gillem, A., & Thompson, C. (2004). Introduction: Biracial women in therapy: Between the rock of gender and the hard place of race. *Women and Therapy, 27*(3/4), 1–18.

Greene, B., & Herek, G. (Eds.). (1994). *Lesbian and gay psychology: Theory, research, and clinical applications (Psychological perspectives on lesbian and gay issues)*. Thousand Oaks: Sage.

Hamilton, J., Jensvold, M., Rothblum, E., & Cole, E. (Eds.). (1995). *Psychopharmacology from a feminist perspective*. Binghamton: Haworth Press.

Herman, J. (1993). *Trauma and recovery* (reprint ed.). New York: Basic Books.

Hill, M. (Ed.). (1998). *Feminist therapy as a political act*. Binghamton: Haworth Press.

Hill, M., & Ballou, M. (1998). Making therapy feminist: A practice survey. *Women and Therapy, 21*, 1–16.

Hill, M., & Ballou, M. (Eds.). (2005). *The foundation and future of feminist therapy*. Binghamton: Haworth Press.

Hill, M., & Rothblum, E. (Eds.). (1996). *Classism and feminist therapy: Cutting costs*. Binghamton: Haworth Press.

Jackson, L., & Greene, B. (Eds.). (2000). *Psychotherapy with African American women: Innovations in psychodynamic perspectives and practice*. New York: Guilford Press.

Jordan, J. (Ed.). (1997). *Women's growth in diversity: More writings from the Stone Center.* New York: Guilford Press.

Jordan, J., Hartling, L., & Walker, M. (Eds.). (2004). *The complexity of connection: Writings from the Stone Center's Jean Baker Miller Training Institute*. New York: Guilford Press.

Jordan, J., Stiver, I., Miller, J. B., Caplan, A., & Surry, J. (Eds.). (1991). *Women's growth in connection: Writings from the Stone Center.* New York: Guilford Press.

Josselson, R. (1995). *The space between us: Exploring the dimensions of human relationships*. Thousand Oaks: Sage.

Kaschak, E. (1992). *Engendered lives: A new psychology of women's experience*. New York: Basic Books.

Kessler, S. (1998). *Lessons from the intersexed*. Rutgers: Rutgers University Press.

Leeder, E. (2006). Inside and out: Women, prison and therapy: A feminist dialogue on challenging correctional discourse. *Women and Therapy, 29*(3/4), 1–8.

Lerman, H., & Porter, N. (Eds.). (1990). *Feminist ethics in psychotherapy*. New York: Springer Publishing.

Miller, J. B. (1976). *Toward a new psychology of women*. Boston: Beacon Press.

Miller, J. B., Jordan, J., Stiver, I., Walker, M., Surrey, J., & Eldridge, N. (2004). Therapists' authenticity. In J. Jordan, L. Hartling, & M. Walker (Eds.), *The complexity of connection: Writings from the Stone Center's Jean Baker Miller Training Institute* (pp. 64–89). New York: Guildford Press.

Miller, J. B., & Stiver, I. (1998). *The healing connection: How women form connections in both therapy and in life*. Boston: Beacon Press.

Miller, J. B., Walker, M., & Rosen, W. (Eds.). (2004). *How connections heal: Stories from relational-cultural therapy*. New York: Guilford Press.

Olkin, R. (1999). *What psychotherapists should know about disability*. New York: Guildford Press.

Ratts, M., D'Andrea, M., & Arredondo, P. (2004). Social justice counseling: "Fifth force" in the field. *Counseling Today, 47*(1), 28–30.

Rave, E., & Larsen, C. (1995). *Ethical decision making in therapy: Feminist perspectives.* New York: Guilford Press.

Walker, L. (2000). *Abused women and survivor therapy: A practical guide for the psychotherapist.* Washington, DC: American Psychological Association.

West, C. M. (2002). Battered, black, and blue: An overview of violence in the lives of black women. *Women and Therapy, 25*(3/4), 5–27.

Worell, J., & Remer, P. (2003). *Feminist perspectives in therapy: Empowering diverse women.* Hoboken, NJ: Wiley.

CHAPTER 6

The Practice of Psychotherapy: *Application*

Charity Tabol and Gail Walker

The previous chapter presented a theoretical framework for feminist therapy practice. This chapter demonstrates applications of the core feminist therapy principles reviewed in Chapter 1, including the following: awareness of multiple spheres of influence at work in clients' lives; appreciation of sociostructural contributions to "psychological" phenomena; attention to issues of power and privilege in the therapy relationship; a focus on client strengths and on the communicative or adaptive aspects of perceived "symptoms"; recognition of the need for therapist self-awareness and the judicious use of therapist self-disclosure; the view of therapy as a political act; and concern for social change. These principles are central to feminist therapy regardless of the particular client and her or his identified presenting problems.

With descriptive case examples, we illustrate the divergence of feminist therapy from mainstream approaches (in both process and content); provide new templates for conducting therapy; and inspire the reader to apply existing skills, techniques, and strategies in more egalitarian and collaborative ways. Most any therapeutic technique or strategy can be used in a manner consistent with feminist therapy principles. Attention to sociocultural context and to matters of power in the way the technique or strategy is introduced, implemented, and evaluated in therapy is what differentiates feminist from standard practice. For example, homework is utilized as a strategy in many forms of therapy. Within traditional approaches, homework is typically assigned to the client by the therapist, as a function of the therapist's assessment of what additional or real-world practice (of a new skill or behavior, for example) is needed to enhance the therapy. The client then reports back to, or shows a homework "product" to, the therapist, as a student would to a teacher. To ameliorate the "power-over" aspect of homework, a feminist therapist would instead collaborate with the client on deciding the homework's focus and tasks. The therapist would not "grade" the client, and doing or not doing the homework would be the client's choice. Homework would empower the client by making her or him the agent of change, the doer. Homework, in feminist therapy, does not emphasize proving new "skills" or compliance with the therapist, but instead provides the client with evidence of doing, being, and feeling differently and can be viewed as an exercise in self-care and self-empowerment.

ABBY

Contextualization of the Client and the "Problem"

Contextualization involves both therapist and client working to understand all the external factors and spheres of influence contributing to the client's identity and situation. Thus, it is not just an exercise in conceptualization for the therapist; it is an intervention in its own right. Contextualizing, by reframing the presenting "problem" as one with roots and influences external to the client, is depathologizing and helps to ameliorate the client's shame and self-blame. A client's distress can often be understood as an understandable reaction to oppression and its demoralizing and resource-depleting effects; a symptom may serve to communicate something to someone else about that oppression—including rejection or protest of it; and an exhibited "problematic" behavior may be a learned way of surviving or adapting to a pathological relationship or system (the latter of which will be a familiar concept to couples therapists and family therapists). In feminist therapy, the therapist not only holds these realities in mind, but also assists the client—through education, support, and validation—in naming, revealing, and challenging external sources of oppression. Contextualizing provides the client with information about the often-invisible stratifications and means of coercion and oppression in our culture, and this information is empowering and permits new choices. The client comes to examine how she or he is affected by privilege, power, and internalized norms and expectations (the "shoulds" and other messages transmitted through various interpersonal and cultural mediums). What was once accepted as "fact" or "just the way it is" or "the only option" can instead be seen as a social construction, a cultural prescription, or one option among several others. Depathologizing the client and her or his distress in this way, and helping to mobilize the client's energy to identify and choose new ways of responding to oppressive dynamics, is one characteristic of feminist therapy.

This process can begin with the therapist creating a mental grid to map the client's "ecology"—the multiple contexts in which the client is embedded, including family, intimate partnerships and other relationships, neighborhood or community, school or workplace, geographical region, and broader social, economic, and political structures; as well as cultural variables such as race or ethnicity, gender, religion, sexual orientation, age, ability or disability status, and class and socioeconomic status. Although many therapeutic approaches consider an individual's "cultural coordinates" when formulating problems and devising interventions, some stop short at recognizing culture's impact on values, customs, and beliefs—missing the subtler issues of power and stratification in society.

The grid situates the client at the center of multiple spheres of influence and intersecting and overlapping identities, all of which contribute to the client's ways of thinking, feeling, relating to others, and generally viewing and being in the world. The grid helps to identify power hierarchies in the client's life; relationships and structures in which power (relational, social, economic, and political) is unequally distributed; and potential sources of oppressive messages and biased expectations. The grid can thereby uncover what is invisible at first glance and what might otherwise be overlooked in the therapy office. A feminist therapist has, through training and education, previous knowledge of what is made invisible in our culture at large—and in particular knowledge of how women, people of color, and members of the GLBT community are marginalized—but also needs to learn from the particular client about what is downplayed or minimized in the client's immediate environment or groups. The grid is a mental framework for tracking starting points and directions for the therapy.

In Abby's case, the therapist's mental "grid" would include consideration of Abby's overlapping and intersecting identities as an African American, a woman, a college graduate, an individual raised in a small town who now lives in an urban environment, a child of divorced parents and a stepfamily, and a survivor of childhood sexual abuse. It would include consideration of her current neighborhood and community, socioeconomic status, employment setting and status, relationships, and other affiliations and group memberships. While exploring with Abby her identified reasons for seeking therapy at this time (recurring worry about leaving her condo door unlocked, worry about her mother's distress, worry about running out of time to have children), the feminist therapist would hold certain diagnostic and clinical constructs in mind—such as the possibility of benzodiazepine abuse, the possible presence of a biologically mediated anxiety disorder, and the possibility that Abby's preoccupation with her condo door being locked is a manifestation of hypervigilance and suggestive of PTSD specifically. However, the feminist therapist would not stay locked in "medical model" thinking (and its emphasis on individual deficits) and would also consider how the sociocultural variables and contexts just named have contributed to or interacted with these presenting concerns. For example, Abby's worry about the condo being unlocked may in part represent more generalized fears for her safety as a woman living alone. She may accurately perceive her neighborhood as unsafe, particularly if she is aware of racial tensions or anti–African American sentiments in her community, or if she has recently been harassed or targeted in some way. In other words, the belief that the world is an unsafe place, or that extra precaution is necessary, should not be dismissed as invalid or distorted, particularly when held by members of groups who are disempowered and disproportionately victimized. These factors might be overlooked by a therapist of another orientation, whose first inclination may be to conceptualize the recurring worry and checking behavior as related to an unresolved psychic conflict, or as a symbolic representation of some unexpressed fear or need, or (reductionistically) as a behavioral stimulus–response pairing that needs to be broken down and extinguished.

Further, regarding Abby's other presenting concerns, the therapist might consider, and at some point explore with Abby, whether there are external messages (from friends, family, the media, or the community at large) that shaped her belief about someday having children (or belief that women should have children) or her beliefs or feelings about being alone and not in a relationship (and what it means to feel she is "running out of time"). The therapist would also consider any links between Abby's current worries about her mother and worry Abby might have had in the past regarding disclosure of the sexual abuse to her mother, and what role gender and power dynamics within the family have played in each set of worries.

Abby's therapist might also consider how her sexual abuse history, compounded by the secrecy that both perpetrator and society encourage surrounding abuse (particularly abuse of women and children), may contribute to her level of general anxiety, her specific worries, and her use of substances to erase her feelings. It would be valuable to explore with Abby her personal knowledge of African American culture, small-town culture, and the "culture" of her family to better understand what she learned at various stages of life about gender and race dynamics, power in relationships, and her own personal power. It might also be necessary to validate Abby's lack of power as a young child, in service of exonerating any guilt or self-blame she may feel for the abuse and rightly placing blame on her stepfather and on a culture that devalues women and children, particularly women and children of color, and perpetuates objectification and exploitation of their bodies. In addition, Abby and her therapist might consider to what extent her anxiety is grounded in the overall loss of personal agency and sense of helplessness that so often result from childhood trauma and abuse.

Abby's anxiety could also be exacerbated by her feeling pressure to look capable and achieve success as an African American woman who is college-educated, in the face of stereotypes to the contrary and institutionalized racism and sexism. In addition, women not only face pressures to perform well academically and on the job, but also are judged on their ability to form and maintain relationships and to carry out caretaking and domestic responsibilities as a wife and mother. Recognition of these and other internalized expectations or norms that may contribute to her anxiety could help Abby to personalize her difficulties less and, along with treating her reaction to such pressures as understandable and common and treating the pressures themselves as the "disordered" element of the equation, thus further serve to depathologize Abby and her situation and empower her to see, question, challenge, and even reject some of these pressures.

Within feminist therapy, contextualization does not apply only to the client and her or his presenting issues. The feminist therapist would necessarily apply a similar grid to herself or himself to assess and explore her or his own sociocultural contexts, identities, beliefs, values, worldview, and level of privilege and how these might affect her or his ability to connect with and work effectively with any client. There are likely areas of shared experience and areas of divergent experience, both categories of which must be considered. In the case of Abby—to name but a few considerations—is her therapist African American? A woman? If not, how will the therapist make a connection with Abby across race or gender? The therapist's values, beliefs, and assumptions regarding class, education, substance use, child abuse, family relationships, and sexual relationships must also be examined. For example, does the therapist assume that because Abby imagines herself having children, she is heterosexual? Does the therapist assume that because both the therapist and Abby are college educated, they enjoy equal privilege in the working world or in social contexts?

Therapy Relationship and Process

Feminist therapy asserts that the process, not just the content of therapy, is healing. Because much injury is an outcome of the misuse of power, there is a conscious effort to share power in the therapy process, and power is named and discussed as one characteristic of the therapy relationship. This is a core element of feminist therapy. If unchecked, therapy can replicate dominant power dynamics in two ways. In its content, it can enforce cultural norms and shape clients toward adjustment to those norms; in its process, the therapist can exercise continual power over the client by acting as an expert who implements a mechanistic protocol and acts *upon* (as opposed to *with*) a client. Feminist therapy regards the dynamics of how the therapy is conducted as an integral part of the healing and empowering tasks of therapy. Feminist therapists heal clients by guiding the clients toward the same agency during sessions that the clients may be striving to effect outside of session.

The intention in feminist therapy is to "walk with" the client, not "do to" the client. To accomplish this, the therapist works to demystify, collaborate, share power, and otherwise shape the process to be congruent with the principles of feminist therapy (one of which is client empowerment). To demystify the therapy process, a feminist therapist strives for transparency in her interactions with the client, by being careful to use nontechnical language, explaining exactly how therapy can help to address the client's areas of concern, explaining fully the ground rules and process of how therapy works, and encouraging the client to ask questions. The therapist might articulate, in the course of therapy, "Here's what I'm doing" or "Here's why I'm pressing you about that." There is continuing awareness by the therapist of the times and points at which the client might need clarification, might have valid reservations (not to be interpreted as pathological "resistance"), or might disagree.

In turn, just as she or he encourages the client to ask questions, the feminist therapist also asks the client questions about her or his lived experience, rather than making assumptions or extrapolations based on academic theory, previous clients, or the therapist's own experience (although these sources of information can certainly be held in mind). The feminist therapist's strivings for transparency, as noted previously, extend to the acknowledgment of her or his own areas of limited expertise or experience. By soliciting the client's truth and knowledge, and regarding and engaging the client as the "expert" on her or his own experience (rather than imposing a preconceived framework or assuming an authoritative stance when it comes to the client's life), the feminist therapist shares power, and the process of therapy becomes collaborative and egalitarian (Fletcher, 1999). Importantly, recognizing the client's expertise, sharing power, and respecting the client's voice mean that the feminist therapist also honors the client's stated concerns or identified "problems," rather than taking over the formulation of goals for, and process of, therapy based on suspicions of the client's denial or minimization of other issues or based on knowing better what the "real" goals should be.

In addition to asking questions about the client's outside experience, background, and goals or concerns relevant to therapy, the feminist therapist will also likely inquire about the client's experience in therapy—how the client feels about a cultural difference between them, for example, or whether the therapist's choice of words in a given moment was experienced as disempowering or stigmatizing. Sharing vulnerability in this way and in other clinically appropriate ways is a form of sharing power. Feminist therapy encourages shared vulnerability rather than disowned vulnerability on the part of the therapist. That vulnerability could also take the form of therapist self-disclosure about some aspect of her or his own lived experience, if it were apparent that such information would be helpful to the client.

A higher octave of shared vulnerability could occur with the therapist sharing in the moment about her responses in that session. There might be an instance where the therapist perceives that a response (or lack of response) might have been a clinical error. In that moment, the therapist can name the concern: "it feels like my comment wasn't helpful and might have had a bad effect on you," or "I think I just made an error," or "just now my silence seems to have created distance between us." This gives the client power. The therapist could go on to model apology and work through the unintentional hurting. Apology by a therapist shares power and prioritizes the relationship over the power of the role. Power sharing and the goal of empowerment also commit the feminist therapist to recognizing, naming, and engaging with the clients' strengths, skills, capabilities, and possibilities (rather than emphasizing areas of need, deficit, vulnerability, or futility, as some orientations do).

In Abby's case, it is clear why sharing power in therapy would be especially critical. Part of Abby's history, and injury, has involved being silenced, keeping parts of herself out of relation, and being denied ownership of her own body. Part of Abby's healing would therefore involve having voice, ownership, and encouragement to share her hidden parts now, in the therapy relationship (or else the therapy, as previously noted, will replicate the oppressive power dynamics she has already experienced, which may in turn reinforce perceptions of others being untrustworthy and exploitative, or herself as lacking worth or agency—and thus make therapy yet another unsafe and marginalizing space).

Sharing power in Abby's therapy would also involve allowing her to frame and define the problem. Upon discovering Abby's sexual abuse history, some might identify it as the key issue and label a different view by Abby as resistance or denial. Her expressed anxieties and sources of concern might be trivialized or interpreted as somehow symbolically representative of the "real" issue by mainstream therapists. A feminist therapist would not make such assumptions and interpretations, but would respect Abby's definitions (the therapist also would not ignore the reality of the abuse, might identify it as potentially of importance, and would extend the invitation to bring it into the therapy—but above all would respect Abby's decision in the matter).

A feminist therapist could also share power and vulnerability by asking Abby how she feels about coming to therapy in the first place and how she feels about having a therapist of a different race or gender (if that were the case). A feminist therapist would also share responsibility for the direction and process of therapy with Abby. Once Abby's concerns and goals had been identified and clarified, a feminist therapist versed in different therapeutic techniques might explain and discuss the options with Abby (including matters of rationale, what the technique would "look like" in practice, and the pros and cons based on the therapist's knowledge of Abby), invite questions, and solicit her input as to which to choose and why. In collaboration with Abby, the therapist might identify the circumstances that would allow Abby to feel interested and safe in trying each technique. The therapist might ask, "If you might want to try this, are you aware of anything that could make you feel safer as we try?" Most good therapists customize the therapy process to some degree to enhance what works with a specific client. However, a feminist therapist would take it further by emphasizing client choice in determining which approach seems best at any given time.

Other key aspects of the therapy process and relationship for Abby might be the way her body and her sexuality are discussed and—relatedly—the identification and showcasing of strengths and joyful possibilities. With regard to the former, Abby's previous discussion or consideration of her bodily experience may have cast her body as the site of violation, symptom, and disempowerment (and her silencing in childhood cast it as a site of shame and secrecy). Thus, her body may have been ignored as a source of strength, well-being, or pleasure. Similarly, based on her history, Abby may hold only negative views of her sexuality, which may have been reinforced by further exposure to cultural scripts portraying women's sexuality as being for men's benefit and exploitation. Mindfully discussing in therapy Abby's body and sexuality in ways that affirm her ownership, agency, and wholeness and that identify alternative "relationships" with, and possibilities for, her body and sexuality would therefore likely have a healing and empowering effect. To achieve this, the feminist therapist might incorporate expressive or body-centered techniques that reconnect Abby with her body, might incorporate bibliotherapy or use of films and images for discussion, would be mindful of including empowering and strength-centered language when discussing Abby's sexuality, and might ask Abby to identify role models that represent a vitality of sexual expression that Abby imagines for herself.

On a related note, Abby's therapist should attend to and centralize Abby's strengths more generally in the process and direction of therapy. As previously noted, whereas the medical model and mainstream approaches to therapy emphasize what is sick in the individual, feminist therapy looks for areas of strength and areas for further growth and learning. Rather than discussing the use of alcohol and medication in shaming or pathologizing terms, for example, a feminist therapist might validate that these choices represented Abby's best efforts to cope with difficult emotions given the resources available to her, but also provide information and education to Abby on the addictive nature of benzodiazepines and the potential consequences of continued use or a continued pattern of stopping and starting erratically (i.e., the dangers of withdrawal). The therapist should also highlight Abby's resilience in surviving her childhood experience, giving up alcohol, managing significant anxiety to accomplish substantial goals, and seeking help when she needed it (to name but a few signs of strength). Recognizing and naming Abby's strengths not only is validating and encouraging, but also arms her with an arsenal of resources she will trust to draw from when responding to future challenges.

Beyond Individual-Level Interventions

Feminist therapists recognize that individual-level interventions are not always sufficient (because the sources of oppression, disconnection, and psychological harm or injury may remain in the client's life, or in the culture at large, and because experiences outside of individual therapy are what may be most healing for the client). The feminist therapist's sharing of power sometimes extends to giving up some power associated with the traditional "therapist" role or power over the intervention entirely, by adopting nontraditional roles (identifying sources of instrumental support or other resources in the community, or contacting an institution to advocate for the client, for example) or by referring clients to other types of interventions. Sharing power might lead a therapist to emphasize that healing can come from immersion in nurturing and encouraging peer relationships or in community settings rather than the mental health system and to identify or locate those potential sources of support. The contextual grid constructed early in the therapy may be helpful in this regard. By explicitly attending (with the therapist's guidance) to the cultural frameworks in which she or he is embedded, the client may discover alliances, resources, and potentially supportive networks she or he had not previously considered.

Abby might find 12-step programs, abuse survivor support groups, women-centered Internet forums, or other collectives or supports (perhaps within the African American community, or perhaps involving a religious, political, or other affiliation) helpful. She might find an intervention involving her and her mother—and repairing their communication and connection—more healing and enriching than individual therapy. She might at some point feel empowered by helping other survivors through volunteerism, by becoming a victims' advocate, or by lending her voice to cultural and political discussions of child abuse or exploitative gender and power dynamics. The idea would not be to authoritatively prescribe these activities to Abby, but to raise her awareness of their existence and of the possibility that individual therapy is not the only, or even necessarily the best, medium for healing, growth, or empowerment.

In feminist therapy, clients are potentiated to utilize their own resources and the resources of their cultures and to connect with others and be a resource to them. In addition, feminist therapists are potentiated to engage in advocacy, activism, and other methods of social change outside the therapy room, to name and challenge systemic and structural inequalities and sources of oppression. Feminist therapists recognize that without macro-level change, cultural "sicknesses" will persist, and individuals will continue to suffer from exposure to, and internalization of, them. Thus, Abby's therapist might engage in the types of advocacy and activism noted previously or be otherwise politically and socially active (through writing, community and grassroots organizing, or support of certain legislative or policy efforts, perhaps) in support of victims' rights and the identification and remediation of oppressive relational and cultural dynamics and forces.

ANNA AND SERGEI

Contextualization of the Client and the "Problem"

In Anna and Sergei's case, the therapist's mental grid of their overlapping and intersecting contexts and identities would be multilayered and complex. The grid would include such factors as their culture of origin (which would provoke consideration of differences between their social, political, and economic experiences in Russia and those in the United States), as well as their current level of acculturation or assimilation and issues of language. The grid would also include culturally prescribed gender roles and how each member of the couple adheres to or departs from them; their religious identity; their employment status; their current urban environment and its level of safety; their degree of connection to or disconnection from family and other supports; their child's illness; and Sergei's injury or disability status. Critically, the grid would also identify multiple macro-level forces and structures that serve as sources of oppression, isolation, and alienation for the couple, including a deficient and morally bankrupt health care system, lack of job security and workers' rights for skilled craftspeople and hourly wage earners, political disempowerment of immigrants and anti-immigrant sentiment and discrimination in our culture, the lack of affordable child care and housing in much of the United States, the lack of adequate social and community assistance more generally, and a host of related and resulting economic and social pressures and inequalities that are often rendered invisible within the dominant culture.

Other macro-level forces of relevance are those that most directly brought Anna and Sergei to therapy—specifically, the involvement of social services and the power over Anna and Sergei that social services has exercised by referring them for therapy (despite finding, assuming an initial investigation was made, that their children were not actually being injured or mistreated). Consideration of all these contextual factors compels us to face that despite all of the aforementioned societal ills and deeply entrenched disparities presenting barriers to their and their children's well-being, it is Anna and Sergei who have been identified as embodying the "problem" (and thus it is they who have been referred for an intervention).

Constructing the grid helps the feminist therapist to see that there is far more going on for Anna and Sergei than just "stress," "worry," and marital arguments and that in light of the obstacles they face to taking care of and providing for their children, they are far from abusive or irresponsible parents. A therapist not versed in, or open to, contextualizing the problem in this way may see Anna and Sergei's needs in terms of "stress management," better communication or conflict-resolution skills, or better parenting skills. A traditional cognitive-behavioral therapist might target patterns in Anna and Sergei's thinking that could be labeled "self-defeating" or otherwise interfering with more effective coping or problem solving. Such areas of focus might serve a minimally helpful function, by providing Anna and Sergei with some surface-level strategies to alleviate intense anxiety or curb worry or anger just enough to avoid or truncate an argument—but this would still leave larger systemic and structural problems unaddressed and thus would leave Anna and Sergei open to continued (and likely, escalating) struggle and distress.

In addition to benefiting the therapist's understanding, contextualization of Anna and Sergei's situation should proceed with them, in the therapy, which constitutes a depathologizing intervention. The therapist should explore with Anna and Sergei their perceptions of their difficulties (which may include self-blame and resultant feelings of shame) and can slowly work outward to incorporate identifications and clarifications of the roles of larger systems and structures in their difficulties, thus ameliorating the internalization of blame. The therapist can normalize for Anna and Sergei their feelings of anxiety, anger, and powerlessness as predictable effects of being at the mercy of powerful and oppressive systems.

Ameliorating shame and self-blame in this way might have additional healing effects for Anna and Sergei. When individuals feel shame, they are often more likely to avoid others or hide their vulnerabilities rather than to reach out for help. By shifting their understanding of the sources of their difficulties (to the external, rather than the internal), the therapist may also increase the likelihood that Anna and Sergei would consider reaching out to others in their community for instrumental help, advocacy, or emotional support. Certain strands of feminist theory, such as relational cultural theory, stress that forming and maintaining relationships or connections with others is the basis of psychological health (Miller & Stiver, 1997). Isolation and disconnection from others is seen as predisposing people to distress. Relational connections are especially critical for individuals in marginalized groups, including Anna and Sergei, whose vulnerability is heightened by their disempowered status and their isolation. Individuals who straddle or negotiate two or more cultures or group allegiances, as Anna and Sergei do, may also be particularly vulnerable to feeling isolated or disconnected. This would be important to highlight for the couple in therapy, to further contextualize their distress.

Contextualization of Anna and Sergei's distress, both in the therapist's mind and as discussed with the couple in therapy, might also include a consideration of gender role socialization and how it has contributed to their current level of distress. The therapist may solicit information as to men and women's traditional "roles" in Russia (what qualities and activities are valued and encouraged in each gender, for example) and as to whether Sergei is struggling with additional feelings of shame, guilt, or low self-worth for being out of work and at home with the children, rather than being a "good provider" (whereas, conversely, Anna's distress may be compounded by feeling like a "bad mother" for working day and night and perhaps missing some of her young children's milestones). These feelings may make it difficult for Anna and Sergei to support one another in their new roles and thus may contribute to overall marital strain. The therapist, by bringing these internalized "shoulds" and expectations to light, helps shift some responsibility for the distress to cultural factors and allows for consideration of possibilities beyond the narrow prescribed definition of "the way things should be" when it comes to men's and women's roles and qualities. Ultimately, if this avenue proved a fruitful one, the therapist might enlist Anna and Sergei in an examination of the value and worth of their nontraditional contributions and roles within the family and to demonstrate how their preexisting, self-identified skills, strengths, and sources of pride are relevant to—and can be transferred to—their different roles.

The greater the number of external structures and systems revealed in contextualizing Anna and Sergei's distress, the more opportunities the therapist has for education, resource sharing, and problem solving with the couple. The therapist could depathologize their difficulties with negotiating our health care system by explaining its well-documented structural problems. Anna and Sergei could be provided with practical information on navigating the system and pursuing resources of which they may not have been aware (such as free clinics, Medicaid, or state health insurance for low-income individuals). In addition, the therapist might identify skills that Anna and Sergei have already demonstrated (and further developed) by making a difficult transition and adapting to a new country and demonstrate how these skills could be generalized to the process of navigating other new structures and institutions, including the health care system.

In keeping with the feminist therapy principle of appreciating context and not operating from a position of blind or unexamined privilege, a feminist therapist would also construct a "mental" grid to illustrate her or his own contexts and identities and areas of convergence with or divergence from Anna and Sergei's. For example, if Anna and Sergei's therapist is native to this country, is she or he prepared to connect across the difference between immigrant and nonimmigrant status and the inherently disparate privilege levels? Is the therapist prepared for how her or his gender will result in different levels of comfort for each member of the couple—and how will this be named and addressed in the therapy? Is the therapist, who is likely not reliant on free health care or social assistance, knowledgeable enough about these resources to be of help to the couple, or will research and self-education be necessary?

Therapy Relationship and Process

Although a focus on empowerment of the client *outside* the therapy office often underlies the feminist therapist's efforts to contextualize clients' distress and to educate and inform clients of external resources and new possibilities, these attempts will be empty exercises in the absence of empowerment *inside* the therapy office as well. The client might merely feel talked at or talked down to, and if outside efforts to follow the therapist's advice fail, this could also engender shame and self-blame. The therapy process provides the unique opportunity for clients to be viewed as equal to, and in partnership with, another person and to practice that process of negotiating power. This not only is healing in validating their worth and respecting their personhood, but also acts as a learning experience that promotes a sense of agency and develops skills in power-negotiating and self-advocacy that can be transferred to other contexts. This would be particularly critical for Anna and Sergei, given the systems and institutions they are attempting to navigate.

If one wound that Anna and Sergei bring to therapy is having felt powerless and ashamed and repeatedly having had things done to them (as their experience suggests may be the case), the therapy must not replicate this. Here again we see the value of contextualizing the presenting "problem" and the means of referral to therapy. As previously noted, Anna and Sergei did not choose to seek therapy, but were mandated through the intervention of social services. A feminist therapist, mindful of their means of entry into therapy (i.e., starting from a doubly disempowered position, both as the client entering the "expert's" domain and as not having made the free choice to be the client in the first place), should focus on encouraging them to choose how they define the problem and on collaborating with the couple to identify what interventions they would find most helpful. Although ready to provide practical information and suggest direction for the therapy if needed, the feminist therapist recognizes that this readiness does not trump the client's wishes or the healing effects of affirming the client's voice and sharing power in the relationship. Further ways to share power in the therapy would involve soliciting Anna and Sergei's vision of the "better life" they are seeking—whether in narrative form or through imagery, metaphor, or symbolic representations—rather than assuming what that phrase means on the basis of the therapist's own life experience and value system. Therapy would aim not only to alleviate their immediate distress but also to empower them to continue pursuing their dream. It might also, however, use contextualization to illustrate how Anna and Sergei's original image of life in the United States may have had certain culturally constructed, romanticized elements and to help the couple determine whether the reality of life in the United States is still in line with what they want most for themselves and their children.

Therapy should also attend to, and centralize, Anna and Sergei's strengths—another means of client empowerment. Anna and Sergei have already demonstrated incredible resilience and determination by making the difficult and risky choice to emigrate from Russia and by staying afloat despite many setbacks and the oppressive influence of powerful systems. They have worked very hard in the interest of providing their children with a better life and have not lost sight of this priority. They remain devoted to one another and flexible in their efforts to cope and sustain themselves economically. They have managed to make some friends in their neighborhood despite having little time to do so and despite barriers of cultural difference and subsequent prejudice. The therapist might emphasize to Anna and Sergei that not many people could have survived their difficult journey at all, let alone with such dignity and with their values and aspirations intact. Calling attention to these areas of strength can inspire or renew clients' hopes, alleviate shame, lead to new understandings of how strengths can be applied, and communicate to the clients their personal power and their status as equal and well-qualified collaborators in the therapy process.

As noted earlier in the chapter, part of sharing power in therapy is sharing vulnerability, which in Anna and Sergei's case might mean acknowledging areas of client expertise and therapist lack thereof. The feminist therapist would therefore readily acknowledge if she or he were uninformed about aspects of the immigrant experience or Russian culture and might solicit the couple's advice about books or resources they would recommend to further the therapist's understanding. The therapist (if not Russian-speaking) should also ask Anna and Sergei if they would prefer a Russian-speaking therapist and refer them appropriately rather than insisting she or he is otherwise "qualified" to treat the couple.

Beyond Individual-Level Interventions

One way feminist therapy would begin to address Anna and Sergei's situation, as already described, would involve inclusion of practical information about various systems and institutions, as well as the pursuit of sources of instrumental support and advocacy. (Such a focus might be familiar to integrative cognitive-behavioral or humanistic therapists, but not—for example—psychodynamic therapists.) There may be immigrant or cultural groups in Anna and Sergei's community or perhaps at a local college or university that could function as a social support network and resource-sharing network for the couple. There might be funds and various forms of social assistance available that were not previously known—something social services may be able to identify, given that they are already aware of the couple's situation. There may be Russian organizations on a state or national level (if not local) that can provide assistance or resources. Because health care, child care, and finding appropriate work for Sergei constitute the couple's major problems at this time, the therapist might work with the couple to help them identify and foster relationships with reliable neighbors who could babysit more regularly or devise a reciprocal arrangement for babysitting in exchange for other needed forms of assistance (perhaps drawing on the couple's existing talents and skills, which include carpentry and baking). There might be a local community center or—importantly—a church (named as something previously important to the couple) where supportive others and instrumental resources could be found. Although it is likely that Anna and Sergei do not have an Internet connection at home, there may be a community center or local library that would offer this resource (which in turn could be utilized to locate relevant job opportunities or other employment resources for Sergei, child care options, or supportive Web sites or chat rooms for the couple—including Russian-language Web sites). Regarding English-as-a-second-language status (and additional "othered" statuses and life experiences, such as immigration, having a disability, or having a child with a chronic illness), connecting with others who share similar identities and obstacles would likely be a relief and a source of empowerment for Anna and Sergei. In addition, it is possible that Sergei's former employer is liable for his injury or that Sergei was entitled to worker's compensation that he never received, and the therapist might assist the couple in contacting legal aid or another service offering free legal information or advocacy. The feminist therapist might discern that these types of resources are all that is needed for Anna and Sergei and would thus not bind them to attending therapy once such resources have been identified and mobilized.

Because feminist therapists recognize the need for social change as well as individual-level interventions, Anna and Sergei's therapist might also pursue advocacy or activism in the area of health care and health insurance, employee rights, affordable child care and housing, and rights and resources for individuals immigrating to the United States. The therapist might join a grassroots network that supports community development efforts; engage in writing, lecturing, or blogging to bring attention to the need for reform of various systems and to expose the predicament of those who are oppressed by such systems; educate colleagues and supervisees about these predicaments; or support legislation and research that address health care disparities and other structural realities that disproportionately hurt the already economically and socially disenfranchised.

SCOTT

Contextualization of the Client and the "Problem"

In contextualizing Scott's situation to understand all the contributing factors, a feminist therapist would consider his family environment, his school and its affiliation with the church, Scott's broader community and region and its climate and values, and cultural factors such as race, gender (and gender socialization), physical appearance, and the socioeconomic status of Scott's family. Viewing the "problem" through these various lenses would reveal, among other things, the contribution of our culture's often-unexamined, rigid, unquestioned gender socialization processes—which make certain behaviors "acceptable" and desirable among girls but not among boys (and vice versa), with deviations from the norm attracting concern and intervention or (at worst) derision, abuse, and harassment (typically, among school-aged children, in the form of boys labeling other boys' behavior as "girly" and wrong when it does not conform to stereotypically male standards).

Contextualization would also reveal whether Scott's family (although apparently egalitarian and tolerant in some ways), church, and—in particular—school appear to support or amplify those socialization processes, in terms of what examples they set (through their own words and behavior; the behaviors they differentially ignore, reinforce, or punish among the students; their construction of classroom activities, hierarchies, and dynamics; and the models they select in the books, films, and other materials utilized in the curriculum). The fact that Scott has been cast as the worst aggressor and referred for therapy, and not the boys who pick on him or "do bad things to girls," is indicative of how deeply entrenched and unquestioned our culture's assumptions about male and female behavior are, and to what extent they have permeated Scott's school. Referring Scott for therapy sends the message that no behavior is as alarming in a child as deviating from gender norms by rejecting undesirable "boyish" behavior (picking on girls, bullying) and making friends outside one's gender. Understanding the contributions of these contextual factors to Scott's lived experience and his referral to therapy allows the feminist therapist to make certain decisions right away about the direction and form that therapy should take, which is further explored in the following section.

Therapy Relationship and Process and Beyond Individual-Level Interventions

Although individual therapy for Scott might be of value as a source of support, validation, and clarification of his current needs, desires, and concerns, the details of this case—once contextualized and once all external factors have entered into consideration—would likely lead the feminist therapist to determine that an intervention on the level of the school would be more appropriate (and that family therapy would also be a useful adjunct to the school intervention, but not the sole modality of intervention given that the family's functioning appears quite healthy). Focusing on Scott alone would perpetuate the notion that the "problem" resides exclusively in him, when in fact he is described as affectionate, sensitive, and helpful and as having friendships (with girls), having a range of interests and activities he enjoys, and doing well in school. It is only in certain contexts that he acts disdainfully or aggressively toward others, and this appears in direct relation to their hurtful behavior toward him and toward others he considers his friends.

That said, a feminist therapist, in service of empowering Scott, might talk with him about what would feel best to him and what, if anything, he would like to change about his situation. Would he like to learn the culture of boys (which could be accomplished through books or films as well as discussion or observation of the boys in his own class) and visit there occasionally? Would he prefer skills for responding to bullying without a goal of befriending boys? Both? Teaching Scott how to make friends with boys (perhaps by identifying an activity of shared interest, or identifying the boy most "like him" in his classroom as a starting point, and then generalizing the social skills he exhibits in his friendships with girls to ways of engaging with this boy) can empower him to have another tool to use when he wants to; however, prescribing that he should be friends with boys and not with girls reinforces and perpetuates oppressive cultural constructs that hurt both boys and girls. The therapist might also utilize Scott's positive relationship with his father as one way of educating him about the different kinds of boys in this world, giving him hope that there may be some—who share the qualities of his father, for example—who are not hurtful and who are worth knowing and being friends with. The therapist might identify activities where Scott and his father could engage with other boys and their fathers in a safe, supervised environment, as an initial foray into the world of boys (not all of whom will behave like those he has experienced at school).

Note that the feminist therapist's method of approaching the "problem" and engaging with Scott differs markedly from that of a behavior therapist or psychoanalytic therapist. A behavioral therapist might construct a reinforcement schedule in consultation with Scott, his parents, and the school—a star for every day Scott did not trip another child, or some other reward identified by Scott as personally meaningful. This intervention does not contextualize the undesirable behavior as embedded in culture. Similarly, a psychoanalytic approach might use play therapy to reveal Scott's "conflicts" and explore his views of gender, but this type of intervention also serves to situate the problem inside Scott, instead of seeing the larger issues of gender role rigidity and the school as a source of cultural indoctrination.

An intervention that is empowering to Scott and that engages him as an equal, collaborative participant in therapy is critical, given that (1) he (by definition, as a child) has entered therapy not of his own volition and in a disempowered status; (2) his suffering and difficulties at school are in direct relation to oppressive dynamics and forces, his reaction to which may represent a way of asserting his own power; and (3) one tool he may currently lack is the ability to assert himself (without aggression) in stressful contexts or in the presence of people he perceives as having power over him. Therapy might provide the opportunity for Scott to practice giving voice to his concerns and advocating for and defending himself without tripping boys or otherwise acting out physically, which currently may represent his only available ways of exhibiting power or protesting unfair abuse of power. Teaching Scott new ways of asserting himself may remove the need for this behavior (or would be one step toward doing so, with changes in the school's environment being the more influential step).

Similarly, focusing on the family unit in isolation would likely have some positive effects, but would be insufficient in scope. Family work might involve sessions with Scott's parents on their own, to identify their own internalized assumptions and expectations about "normative" gender-based behavior and how they may be communicating and reinforcing these assumptions in their home (consciously or unconsciously), as well as sessions with the family as a whole, to observe all the existing dynamics and recognize the value of each family member's contribution to the family's functioning as an overall unit. A feminist approach to family therapy is inherently collaborative. In the process of working with a family where the child is seen as the "problem," a feminist therapist debunks the expectation that the therapist is the only expert and regards the parents as the experts on their child. The therapist would request that the parents collaborate as partners and be transparent, making it explicit how the collaboration works: "I know psychotherapy, and you know your kid. The job can't get done without us working together." In contrast, a non-feminist therapist might elicit information from the parents but then utilize that information to maintain the role as the expert. In feminist therapy, there is collaboration in all aspects—diagnosis, goal-setting and treatment planning, exploring and explaining which modalities might work, evaluating progress toward goals, determining frequency of sessions, and determining when to conclude therapy.

The strengths of Scott's family, including the coparenting approach by his mother and father and both parents' emotional engagement with their children (which may be unusual in their community and is still not the norm in our culture as a whole) and their respectful and gentle manner of addressing the "problem" thus far, without being coercive or punishing to Scott, should be identified and capitalized on. Scott's family appears to be caring, affectionate, and supportive of some "different" forms of play and expression, and these characteristics should be lauded, not pathologized. Scott's behavior might even be reframed as a positive sign of strong moral principles and values, enabled by what his parents have modeled within their home (a more egalitarian approach to parenting and lack of adherence to rigid, unhealthy expectations that one must blindly follow peer example and that men should not show caring or emotion or engage as equals with women). His parents might be encouraged and heartened to know that once freed from certain oppressive contexts, and particularly in adulthood when he has more power to avoid pathological environments, Scott will likely live a more authentic life as a result of his lack of "conformity" at this age. Scott's parents might also appreciate books, films, and testimonials from adult men and women who were also "different" from their same-gendered peers in childhood, or access to other informational resources (or parent groups or support networks) that validate a range of gender expressions in children and reiterate that it is not a cause for alarm or something to be shamed or discouraged.

Although valuable, intervening at the level of Scott's family is insufficient because no matter how supportive and growth-promoting a family environment is cultivated, Scott will have to continually move between this supportive world and one that communicates to him that he and his family are different (and indeed, pathological); that other rules and expectations apply for several hours of each day; and that these other, incompatible rules and expectations will be enforced and condoned by powerful adults. These conflicting messages and expectations can make the world a confusing and stressful place for a 9-year-old. In this sense, stopping with a family intervention might actually set Scott up for greater difficulty.

With regard to intervening at the school level, the therapist might take this on her- or himself or might empower the parents to do so (or some combination of the two approaches). In either scenario, the therapist would likely discuss with Scott's parents how macro-level forces and structures in our culture define gender roles rigidly and how school systems can buy into, and enforce, that culture. Scott's parents might become more empathic toward Scott as they realize just how significant a transition he makes from their house to the classroom. Feminist therapy would empower these parents, by educating, by validating their concerns, and by depathologizing their way of doing things, to have the sense of "rightness" that would motivate them to interact with the school system and advocate for their child.

Once this motivation had been fostered, the therapist or Scott's parents (or all three) might observe a classroom at the school or meet with Scott's teachers and principal (or the school psychologist or counselor, if there is one), to begin a dialogue about Scott's situation and to investigate the school's gendered expectations and assumptions, the books and classroom examples used, and the system of punishments and rewards. Scott's parents, the therapist, or all parties might shift school personnel's attention to the violence and teasing perpetrated by other boys in the class, and if the school is not responsive to addressing this behavior, it may be necessary to transfer Scott to another safer and more tolerant school environment (or classroom, if that is an option within the school and if certain teachers can be identified as more supportive and informed than others). To bolster Scott's parents' readiness to confront school personnel and attempt to initiate changes in the school culture, the feminist therapist might engage in role-playing with them, focus on developing their communication and assertiveness skills, locate other parents in the community who can act as supports and sharers of practical information (or assist Scott's parents in locating them), and identify advocacy resources and information on the legal responsibilities of Scott's school to address intolerance and bullying. Scott's parents, or concerned teachers and school administrators, might be assisted by the therapist in locating relevant Internet resources for addressing gendered bullying in schools, or in locating an outside consultant to help assess and ameliorate the problem.

PRACTICAL CONSIDERATIONS FOR FEMINIST THERAPISTS

A foundation for self-care and consultation may be especially important for feminist therapists. As a result of being more actively engaged in relationships and allowing oneself to share power and vulnerability, the feminist therapist's subjective experience can be different from that of traditional therapists. Peer consultation can avert burnout and compassion fatigue and can provide a forum to review the complexities of sharing power. In addition, because a feminist orientation recognizes the personhood of the therapist more than is the case for mainstream orientations, self-care is an ethical imperative. In addition to collaborating with clients as a way to share power, feminist therapists collaborate with colleagues in peer consultation. Collaboration is essential to share understanding, vulnerability, and support; to avoid hubris; and to do power checks to avoid holding or giving away too much power.

SUMMARY

Feminist therapy is concerned with illuminating the multiple spheres of influence operating in clients' lives (including structural forces that perpetuate the marginalization of nondominant groups), empowering clients in addition to ameliorating their distress, and working for social justice. These concerns are embodied in thoughtful, multilayered conceptualizations of clients and attempts to depathologize clients by identifying the contributions of contextual factors and power disparities to their current situations; in collaborative ways of relating and determining goals and directions for therapy; in demystification of therapy tools and techniques; in therapist transparency and other ways of sharing power and vulnerability; in highlighting client strengths and resilience; and in identifying the need for, and roads toward, social as well as individual change. The intention to empower the client and share ownership of the therapy process is often what distinguishes the use of a "mainstream" technique in feminist therapy from its use in a different form of therapy. In contextualizing the client and her or his presenting "problems," the feminist therapist attends to what is being amplified or minimized and why. The feminist therapist is continually attentive to how power is exercised and negotiated in the therapy relationship, which is crafted to be a key ingredient of the healing work.

Being a feminist therapist involves ongoing self-examination; questioning of one's own embedded and hidden values, beliefs, and assumptions; ongoing consultation; and inclusion of interventions that simultaneously hold multiple aspects of the client's sociocultural contexts and identities in consideration. To fulfill the essence of feminist therapy, the therapist not only focuses on empowerment and change on an individual level, but also reaches beyond the therapy dyad to consider, include, or substitute other levels of intervention and to engage in advocacy, activism, and other forms of social change and to empower clients to do the same.

REFERENCES

Fletcher, J. (1999). *Disappearing acts: Gender, power and relational practice at work.* Cambridge, MA: MIT Press.

Miller, J. B., & Stiver, I. P. (1997). *The healing connection: How women form connections in therapy and in life.* Boston, MA: Beacon Press.

CHAPTER 7

Ethics and Activism:
Theory—Identity Politics, Conscious Acts, and Ethical Aspirations

Eleanor Roffman

INTRODUCTION

Throughout its complex history, feminist therapy practice has been challenged to integrate the concerns of working-class women, lesbians, bisexual and transgendered women, women of color, and disabled women. This integration reflects the ongoing growth and development of feminism and feminist therapy through the evolution of different movements and theoretical orientations. The tensions between women of different classes, races, ethnicities, and sexualities have played a significant role in women's efforts to bring about social change, especially through the field of mental health. Feminism has contributed significantly to the study of morality and ethics and its applications to practice and activism. This chapter contextualizes the role of feminism and race and class within feminist therapy and its relationship to moral inquiry, ethical considerations, and activism.

CONSCIOUSNESS RAISING AS ACTIVISM WITHIN THE WOMEN'S MOVEMENT: THE PERSONAL IS POLITICAL

The early second-wave women's movement, not unlike the first wave, started off as a predominantly white women's movement. Women of color and other women distant from the white middle-class heterosexual norms struggled to have their issues recognized by this movement. Women from the dominant culture emphasized gender, whereas women from oppressed groups urged the white middle-class majority within the women's movement to raise their consciousness not only about their individual situations and relationship to their male counterparts within the dominant culture, but also to their relationship to women of color, lesbians, working-class women, disabled women, and others marginalized by the dominant culture. Older women as well pointed out the ageism within the women's movement.

Throughout the 1980s and 1990s, feminist therapists continued to address issues of sexism, sexual orientation, racism, and classism within theory and practice (Comas-Diaz, 1994; Maracek and Kravetz, 1998). The movement for the empowerment of clients addressed both the power arrangements within the therapeutic relationship and client empowerment within their communities (Adams, 2003).

AGITATION WITHIN THE MAINSTREAM: THE POLITICAL IS PROFESSIONAL

At the height of the second wave of feminism, feminist therapy mirrored what was happening in the surrounding women's movement. In addition to challenging mainstream androcentric psychology and questioning its practice, feminist therapists began confronting psychology's pathologizing of other marginalized groups. As a result, feminist therapists created the tools to empower women in therapy (Ballou, 2005; Maracek & Kravetz, 1998). As feminist therapists became more conscious of the role of context in understanding the life situations of their clients, they became more active in addressing that context.

Today, feminist therapy theory, like women's studies in general, appears to have become more distant from its grassroots origins as it has become more integrated into mainstream educational and clinical institutions (Unger, 1998). Tensions developed between the legitimization of feminist approaches within academe and professional organizations and grassroots community groups, the original foundation of feminist therapy practice. One can ask if feminists are moving into the mainstream or whether the movement into the mainstream by feminists has created greater awareness, thus shifting the boundaries of what is mainstream and what is feminist. Feminists working within mainstream organizations have yielded positive results for women, especially white women. But a drawback to this approach is the weakening of the bonds between professional women therapists and women from grassroots organizations, communities of color, and working-class communities.

IDENTITY POLITICS AND MOVEMENT BUILDING: THE POLITICAL IS PERSONAL

Within the women's movement the examination of the layers of identity and power relationships began as an effort to redress the invisibility of women who differed from the white heterosexual norm. As white women were addressing the essentializing and invisibility of women within academic disciplines, they were also learning that they did not speak for all women. However, as emphasis on differences surfaced in the women's movement, women of color, lesbians, and women from national struggles outside the United States expressed a concern that these differences themselves were becoming essentialized (hooks, 1989).

Habermas, in his "new social movement" theory (1981), examined the difference between social movements before the organized efforts of women, gays, African Americans, and other cultural identity groups. He suggested that earlier labor/capital struggles had focused on material issues, the distribution of wealth under capitalism, and the presence of poverty resulting from this economic system. The "new movements," believed Habermas, were involved with a different process, one that addressed issues of identity and their impact on cultural shifts and changes, and did not emphasize the role of class membership in exploring identities. Identities are expressed in what Habermas called the "lifeworld" (Edwards, 2004), the world of the everyday, the place where our moral and practical considerations are worked through. Feminist therapy addressed the impact of these cultural and personal changes, working with the hurts, insults, and macro- and micro-aggressions placed on the lives of people, especially women, in these "everyday places." However, the focus remained on the import of gender, and as with the struggle around issues of race, feminists did not bring class to the foreground. Gender still remained the organizing feature of feminism, and race and class were secondary. Not unlike the choices made in early feminist organizing, the current choices still reflect the concerns of those in leadership, the mostly white middle-class majority.

Feminist theorists bell hooks (1989) and Tanya McKinnon (hooks & McKinnon, 1996) suggest that the politicization of the self is the path toward theorizing experience. As Laura Brown (1994) suggests, feminist therapy developed as a way to raise feminist consciousness. It brought to awareness that difficulties in living are not just the result of personal vulnerabilities but are a result of the systemic ways that women have been excluded and invalidated by the dominant culture. Addressing issues of power is central to a feminist sociopolitical analysis and a key area of discourse within the practice of feminist therapy. Feminist therapists brought into feminist theorizing and into the therapeutic relationship a multifaceted examination of issues of power: the power within the larger social context, the power assigned to the role of therapist, and the power dynamics within the therapy relationship itself as well as the client's relationship to power personally and politically.

As white feminists challenged the male majority within psychology, women of color and other disenfranchised women challenged the separations created by white heterosexual privilege. Feminist therapists began to make important connections between psychology's pathologizing of women and the pathologizing of other disenfranchised groups. Women of color, lesbians, working-class women, ethnic minorities, and radical women struggled, and still do struggle, to have their voices heard within the larger women's movement and within the feminist therapy community (Comas-Diaz, 1994; Espin, 1994). The multicultural counseling movement developed through the agitation of those marginalized and invisible to the mainstream.

BUILDING ALLIANCES

Interestingly, the multicultural counseling movement has encouraged us to perceive identity development as a process that occurs situationally within experience, benefits from consciousness raising, and builds alliances between people who share the same inquiry and social goals (Cross, 1995; Helms, 1995). Creating allies seems to reflect a level of movement that breaks isolation, fosters new ways of looking at concerns, and provides support for social action. Theoretically and practically, there are opportunities available for feminists to form alliances with other psychological strands that address topics key to the feminist agenda.

Feminists have been instrumental in bringing to the therapeutic encounter a political analysis of power dynamics that affect women in relationships, families, the workplace, the communities in which they live, education, and health care systems. These areas of attention link feminism to critical psychology and liberation psychology.

Critical theory and critical psychology emphasize an examination of power differentials in relationships and seek to balance decision-making power predicated on a set of beliefs centered in concepts of social justice. Habermas (1981) rethought critical theory's Marxist origins and explored critical theory as a vehicle for self-knowledge and self-liberation. He was influenced by psychology and, in turn, influenced psychology. His work encouraged progressive thinkers to frame an understanding of control as a function of internal colonization and to understand its impact on people's daily lives. Habermas and other critical psychologists addressed the importance of embracing people's strengths to bring about systemic change.

Liberation psychology, like feminist and critical psychology, is also derived from a political movement, the liberation theology movement. The liberation theology movement has its roots among the poor in Central and South America and addresses the inequities and injustices of poverty (Martin-Baro, 1994).

Michelle Toomey, a liberation psychologist (1992), suggests that psychology, including the feminist liberal strand, offers reforms of, not rebellions against, basic assumptions that continue to degrade women. She suggests that we need to create a historical context for understanding the ways we are co-opted into androcentric perspectives. For example, she asks why we need to justify the value of empathy in relationships rather than address why it has historically been excluded. Toomey offers liberation psychology as a theory that rejects assumptions about gender, sex, power, and control. Liberation psychology, according to Toomey, is an ecological psychology, one that redefines energy as power, and relationships as mutual exchanges of energy.

Feminist theorizing has attended to similar issues through its focus on issues of gender, culture, and power. A feminist commitment to coalition building provides a model for adherents of these different theoretical orientations to work together and not focus on their own predominance at the risk of not attending to the work of social justice (Ballou, 2005). Feminism has the tools to integrate these strands of thought into the therapeutic process and into the lives of practitioners. Feminism, critical psychology, and liberation psychology encourage practitioners to extend practices beyond the therapy hour and place and to engage in activism and strategies for change.

EMPOWERMENT AS A STRATEGY FOR SOCIAL CHANGE

According to Margot Breton (1994), even when one has experienced individual change and feels empowered cognitively and behaviorally, it is difficult to suggest that one is empowered as long as the changes do not impact socially unjust situations. Breton notes, "the power to name must be accompanied by the power to act" (p. 36). Herrick (1995) suggests that an essential aspect of empowerment for social change is the creation of symmetry of relationships.

As with efforts to introduce ethics as a dynamic changing force (Feminist Therapy Institute, 1999), empowerment is also a changing, transformational process. Radical psychiatry (Steiner & Wycoff, 1975), whose roots are in teaching that politics are central to people's problems, suggests that "rescuing" by therapists maintains oppression and does not empower. The politics of radical psychiatry embraced an understanding of power inequities, one that has been reinforced by feminism. Empowerment is the means by which individuals and groups take charge of their lives and circumstances. Empowerment is a democratizing concept, one that values achieving equality, understanding the impact of policies and actions on one's self as well as on communities.

CLASS: THE INVISIBLE DIVIDE

Therapists who emerge from the working class find themselves needing to acculturate to middle-class values in order to survive within the field. Middle-class values, perspectives, and desires predominate throughout the culture of therapy, especially through the beliefs in individualism, internal locus of control, and the privileging of privacy and upward mobility. Oftentimes, working-class life is romanticized, objectified, and stereotyped in ways that render it unrecognizable to the upwardly mobile working-class woman.

Therapists from working-class origins often find themselves affirmed for their assimilation of middle-class behaviors, including how they look and talk. They are reinforced for their passing as middle class. For these therapists, the acknowledgment of discomfort and the exploration of its origins may be the beginning of consciousness raising. Being uncomfortable is a first step to awareness. Paying attention to this discomfort and valuing one's background in spite of the discomfort can create an opportunity for therapists of working-class background to inform themselves and others. Attending to the dissonance and contradictions created between working-class origins and a middle-class educational and training environment can contribute to a sense of membership, strengthen identity, and lead to coalition-building opportunities. Not unlike biracial people, upwardly mobile working-class feminists can be translators and border crossers.

Reasons that class remains invisible within U.S. society and within therapy practice include the reduction of class concerns to a cultural issue, affirming the ubiquity of middle-class life as normative, and not understanding the role that class plays within capitalism. This last point is vital in that those of us raised in the United States are conditioned not to criticize capitalism, but to accept it. This lack of critical thinking supports capitalism's continuation through inculcation of fear, manufacturing of desire, and support for competition. Not unlike issues of race, issues of class are denied and treated as if they were in the past tense and not core to the distribution of power in capitalistic society. Middle-class therapists and people in general need to challenge the embedded social fear that attending to class differences means giving up something of value and not gaining from the process. Like racism and sexism, dealing with class oppression benefits not only the person most directly affected by it, but everyone.

It would seem that an active inquiry into class differences and their implications could create for the feminist therapist an opportunity to examine what informs her thinking on this issue. Additionally, conversations need to take place across class lines, lines that are hidden and obscured. Not unlike mixed groups of the past that dealt with difficult social issues, class-consciousness groups need to be composed of both working-class and middle-class women. The usual power dynamics need to be challenged, and new arrangements need to be supported.

CLASS ANALYSIS AS A KEY FEATURE OF FUTURE FEMINIST THERAPY ACTIVISM

Nancy Fraser's (2003) presentation on social justice in globalization suggests that pushing class struggles to the background and foregrounding cultural identity issues allows therapy to be a vehicle to avoid confronting the power issues related to the redistribution of wealth. She argues that feminists and other change agents have opted for the dimension of recognition rather than redistribution of wealth. The cultural and political gains of the twentieth-century liberation movements, according to Fraser (2003), have been abandoned for a politics of cultural recognition. As Bernstein (2002) suggests and Fraser emphasizes, feminist therapists need to consider the integration of the concerns of the redistribution of social and economic wealth with the concerns of cultural recognition. Without this integration feminist therapists are unable to engage in what Fraser terms a "two dimensional conception of justice" (pp. 3–4). According to this principle, feminist therapists need to work toward changing the social arrangements that perpetuate inequities. The Feminist Therapy Institute's Code of Ethics encourages the recognition of class differences as it does other issues of diversity but does not reflect on these differences as key to the distribution of wealth and power in U.S. society. The tenets of feminist therapy does the same in that it lists class as an area of diversity and one that intersects with gender oppression.

New social movements have both propelled forward and challenged struggles for social justice. Theorists (Habermas1981; Jaggar 1998; Bernstein 2002; Fraser 2003) suggest that although identity and its collective expression are strengthening, they alone cannot contribute to social justice without attending equally to the institutionalized issues of inequity that accompany identity struggles. Without attention to positions of power and status, it is doubtful that those from subordinated groups will achieve much-needed parity. Those from dominant cultures will continue to maintain control over others' resources, both globally and locally, unless those opposed to this actively address these inequities. So what does this mean for those of us who value the development of a moral feminist position?

FEMINIST MORALITY THEORY

Feminist voices from the both the mainstream and the margins have played a major role in transforming the norms and values of the dominant culture and have been central to the discourse that has challenged white superiority, heteronormativity, and the privileges afforded the nuclear family (Bernstein, 2002). Alison Jaggar (1992) suggests that traditional Western ethics are not concerned with women's rights; disregard women's moral development, considering it lesser than men's; and seem to value only masculine expressions of morality. Virginia Held (1993) claims that we need a feminist moral theory because we live in a society that does not value women's input about morality and because traditional moral theories have not drawn from women's experience. Held suggests that androcentric theories have not adequately acknowledged the role of feelings and have overemphasized the role of reason in developing a moral approach to life struggles and dilemmas. Held (1995) suggests that caring and the moral insights developed from caring relationships cannot be captured in universal principles and that we can look toward relationships that are based on trust as a way to think about morality. Held argues that ethics are based on experience, in particular moral experience. She defines moral experience as conscious acts based on moral positions and suggests that we arrive at these positions through both interior and exterior dialogue (1995).

Held (1995), like Habermas (1981), suggests that we need to value the way experience informs our day-to-day lives and our connections with others. Focusing on experiences of everyday life and on relationships has led feminists to address issues of caring about the self, the other, and the globe (Ballou, Matsumoto, & Wagner, 2002). Consequently, the experience of women is primary to developing moral positions. The experience of those marginalized in society is ever more crucial to incorporate because the perspectives of the privileged are often veiled by their privilege (Held, 1995). This posture can guide us to lifting that veil by consulting and being informed by those who are not obstructed by the veil. We return again to the import of coalitions and primary resources for information. We can ask who is part of the external dialogue required for a balanced view. Abrahams (1992) suggests that by locating problems of everyday life in the range of women's lives, we can demystify the process of domination.

FEMINIST ETHICAL CODES

The transformation of cultural norms requires that political action and process also be transformed. Ethical principles of practice within feminist therapy affirm efforts to travel across divides of race, class, and sexual orientation and bring a more potent consciousness to the work of feminist therapists. Feminist therapy practice and feminist ethics highlight the differences in power and social advantage based on gender and the intersection of gender with race, class, social, political, and economic domination. (Brown & Ballou, 1992; Hare-Mustin & Maracek, 1990). Both feminist therapy and feminist ethics alert feminists to the social construction of dominance and to the accepted notion that domination is a valuable and necessary tool for survival. Feminist codes of ethics such as Brabeck and Ting's tenets of feminist therapy (2000) and the Feminist Therapy Institute (FTI) Code of Ethics (1999, in Appendix B) reflect the efforts of feminists to keep the link between practice and theory alive. Both these codes of ethics emphasize the differences in power and social advantage based on gender and its intersection with race, class, social, political, and economic domination.

Although both codes address issues of oppression and the need for social change, the realities of the society in which we live challenge the impact of these documents. In many situations, it still remains that white middle-class women in the United States are providing services for women who differ from them in terms of social power as determined by race, class, ethnicity, and sexual orientation. How do we change this reality and bridge the values expressed in the tenets of feminist therapy and the FTI Code of Ethics with feminist therapy practice? How do codes of ethics such as the FTI code (1999) address the intersection of everyday life and feminist therapy?

Challenging the realities that create injustices and taking steps to advocate for change are embedded in the FTI code and tenets of feminist therapy (Brabeck & Ting, 2000). Both codes provide parameters for developing an ethics of care by addressing injustices and noting the role of action in confronting the challenges of living within patriarchy, especially as it is relevant to the practice of mental health counseling. The FTI's preamble encourages an understanding of social power through a feminist lens, one that acknowledges the ubiquity of power inequities and the possibilities for feminist therapists to be influenced by oppressive forces. It notes the value of ongoing dialogue to address these influences. The guidelines are divided into five areas: cultural diversities and oppressions, power differentials, overlapping relationships, therapist accountability, and social change.

How can these guidelines promote activism? In the FTI code's first section on cultural diversities and oppressions, the therapist is encouraged to be mindful of the impact of current practices of health care, the meanings of her multiple layers of identity, and the need to educate oneself with regard to dominant and nondominant differences. One could say that this section addresses awareness and its impact on practice, a call for a level of understanding of differences within therapeutic relationships. The second section of the FTI code addresses power differentials and encourages the therapist to be mindful of power differences between the client and the therapist. Section 3 delves more deeply into the therapist–client relationship and addresses multiple relationships within care delivery systems as well as the need to protect the boundaries between therapist and client, especially in regard to sexualized relationships with clients or former clients.

Section 4 of the FTI code addresses professional accountability, realms of competence, continuing education, supervision, and self-care. Finally, Section 5 addresses the fluidity of social change, the role of access to technology, and the responsibility of the therapist to be an agent of change, politically as well as professionally. As we see, the first three sections deal with the therapist and her client relationships as well as her responsibilities to herself and her clientele. The last two sections deal with external accountability and possible avenues for change. The change that is addressed is reformist change, ways to reform inequities within systems. Reformism is significant and important but only a beginning step to providing aspirations and visions for activism. The code presents issues of power within the framework of a consumer rights movement.

This perspective does not offer ways to change the power differential that the code seeks to address.

Brabeck and Ting's tenets (2000) also address five major themes. How do these themes embrace a call to activism? The first theme addresses an ethics of care and nurturance, subjective knowing, and a critique of individualism. The second theme attends to women's subjective experience and relational skills and the attributes of women related to biologically based experiences. It also addresses the need to change unjust structures and oppressive practices and attitudes. The third theme cautions us against privileging the issues of women from the dominant culture as exemplified by standpoint theory—that is, seeing an experience as interpreted by women from their placement within hierarchies that classify and rank them in terms not only of gender but also of class, race, sexuality, and other aspects of identity. The fourth theme asks feminists to critique power hierarchies, including one's position within hierarchies of power. The discussion of this theme cautions us not to engage in a radical relativism but to appreciate the complexities of context and the power dynamics within that context. The fifth theme addresses the relationship between ethics and action. It suggests that it is a feminist responsibility to take action to redress injustices and change systems and if that does not work, to address the injustices within systems. In this section we are cautioned about the individualistic nature of early theories on care and nurturance as well as their apolitical nature. These five overarching themes also have a trajectory of understanding. They begin with the implications inherent in the denial of women; the invisibility, distortion and oppression of women; and how the recognition of women and women's experience can lead us to enriching ways of understanding morality. This is followed by the recognition of the interlocking relationships between forms of oppression and the distortion that occurs when the multiplicities of identity and oppression are not addressed. These codes differ in that the FTI code is more directly addressing therapists and the Brabeck and Ting tenets are addressing a larger audience of feminist academics, researchers, and practitioners. Although both documents cite social class as an issue of power and diversity, they do not address the realities that social class plays within the professions and within communities. Both the FTI code and the tenets of feminist therapy acknowledge the struggle between self-interest as a member of a guild (the practice of feminist therapy) and the need to change the system that supports the guild's practice. Feminist consciousness is key to feminist therapy. Class consciousness is key to examining the distribution of wealth and the inequities and injustices that exist as a result of the power maintained by those who have the wealth. A sharper focus in ethical codes needs to be developed around issues of class and parity of participation (Fraser, 2003) as a way to strengthen feminist activism within the practice of therapy.

APPLICATION OF ETHICS TO FEMINIST THERAPY

Examining political action in everyday life as a behavior involves examining values, resources, beliefs, and expectations. A feminist conception of political action involves an examination of the complexities of power dynamics. As Abrahams (1992) points out, the political acts of those who have no political power are often ignored, as evidenced by the dismissal of black women as role models for white women. A feminist ethic is one that does not accept a monolithic women's perspective and that instead includes the standpoints of women of color, lesbians, poor women, and challenges the dominant paradigms that maintain the status quo.

Although there are many ways to examine ethics from a feminist multicultural perspective, feminists generally agree that the starting point is the everyday lives of women. A multicultural feminist perspective is one that examines not only the nature of oppression in everyday lives, but the sources of this oppression (Sparks & Park, 2002). As feminist therapists, we need to be conscious of our worldviews and the impact of our own socialization in the roles we play in other people's lives.

THERAPIST AS ACTIVIST

Rethinking the role of the therapist as activist requires that we reexamine the notion of activism. Activism has traditionally been perceived in androcentric terms as political action in the public sphere (e.g. lobbying, belonging to professional groups, and addressing institutional systems). A feminist perspective on activism is one that connects the experience of the individual's everyday life to the systemic structures that maintain social control. Abrahams (1992) makes the point that examining political action in everyday life requires a shift in thinking. Political action needs to be considered as a constructive behavior, one that requires skills of negotiation and collaborative thinking and acting and an ability to analyze power. If we consider activism as a learned behavior rather than a place (the public sphere), we are better able to focus our energies as therapists both within the therapeutic relationship and within other activist activities. If we consider the complex relationships between the positions people occupy in interlocking systems of power (race, gender, class) and the activities they engage in to negotiate power, then we are better equipped to strategize and assess how to support positive change. This thinking deconstructs power relations and enables a better sense of appreciation for what it takes for so many people to navigate the struggles and hardships of everyday life. Feminist therapists must recognize the contradiction of their therapeutic role. Their relationships with their clients begin with the assumption that the therapist is the "knowing one." Yet a goal of feminist therapy is to value the "knowing" of the client by both therapist and client. Additionally, the goal of feminist therapists is to empower their clients to act on their own behalf and, in so doing, see themselves as activists for social change.

The FTI Code of Ethics and Brabeck and Ting's tenets of feminist therapy encourage us to guide our practice by attending to the lived experience of women, to understand the historical context and relativity of theory, especially in light of the multiple realities that shape women's lives. They remind us of the necessity of letting go of androcentric biases, and most importantly of seeing our work as action directed.

How do the values expressed within these codes guide us toward activism, a process that differs from action in that activism requires a commitment to engage in organized efforts to address social injustices? Early feminist awareness of domestic violence, incest, child abuse, and the impact of trauma on women's lives led to the development of an activism that shaped current feminist institutions and practices. What seems to be required as we embrace the agenda of the twenty-first century is a continuing commitment to what social workers began more than a century ago—that is, focusing on the person–situation paradigm. In this historical paradigm, however limited by concepts or race and culture, social workers understood problems in living as connected to people's social situations. It seems that an aid in strengthening the bond between feminist therapists and the social justice issues of our time is a refreshed examination of inclusiveness. Understanding more clearly the gender, culture, and class gaps in our society will promote greater efforts to activism.

However, another important issue that needs to be raised is how to bring these codes to therapists and therapists in training. It seems that we need to address curricula in graduate training and clinical training sites and the teachers and clinicians who work with students. Additionally, we need to find ways to continue talking about these issues in forums that engage the professionals as well as in venues that engage grassroots activists working with women in varied settings.

CONCLUDING REMARKS

Creating nondominant dialogues, respecting and attending to the activities of everyday life, emphasizing collaborative alliances, and addressing the issues that keep us apart from those with whom we work or want to work are part of an ongoing process that wrestles with issues of power and control. Understanding the differences between a feminist perspective and a gender-dichotomized approach to life's difficulties is necessary to push forward an agenda based on pluralism, justice, and care.

We are not dealing with the same conditions that fostered our movement in the earlier days of the women's movement. We are dealing with a practice of psychology that creates greater barriers between feminist therapists and their clients. For example, shelters need to meet the requirements of regulatory institutions that often do not demand community engagement. Managed care means that people do not manage their own health care. Regulatory institutions and licensing boards do not encourage or recognize activism as a goal. Educational institutions, in their efforts to provide marketable training, seldom focus on activism as a valued aspect of therapist training. This is not to say that standards of care are uninvited, but it appears that activism has been removed from the landscape of education, within both therapy training and the ongoing practice of the profession. As feminist therapists, we need to reclaim activism as essential to our practice and integrate it within our behavior and in our guidelines for best practices.

Feminist ethics come from a relationship to the feminist movement that is foremost a political movement, a new social movement, one directed not only toward issues of policy and law, but also to other forms of identity. Activism is the result of acting on the conditions that shape these realities. A feminist activism is one that engages with thinking about the multiplicities of identity and taking action for social justice. Feminist therapists are encouraged to play an active role in critiquing the power arrangements of social class within their lives as well as in the lives of their clients. We need to encourage each other to see activism as a desirable behavior to be integrated into our lives and the lives of those we touch.

A feminist therapy practice is one that it is informed by women's positionality as second-class citizens. This second-class status has not meant that issues of race, class, sexuality, and so on were immediately understood and considered, but attention to these issues did promote the caring, empathy, and mutual respect necessary to bring about dialogue and agitation for social change. Understanding the experiences of everyday life is primary to developing a moral perspective and creating ethical guidelines for feminist therapists. Women, so long the healers in multiple societies, have taken on reshaping ethics and activism. Feminist codes of ethical practice are dynamic, informed by women's lived experience, and consequently fluid and open to change. Our involvement in their evolving changes requires us to be involved in the organizations that create and support ethical codes. We can best inform our organizations by attending to the social conditions that bring people to therapy and to the impact of these conditions on the daily lives of those with whom we choose to work and build alliances. We are most credible and effective as agents of change when we emphasize the political dynamics that create the divides as well as the alliances shaped by class, race, and gender.

REFERENCES

Abrahams, N. (1992). Towards reconceptualizing political action. *Sociological Inquiry,* 62(3), 335–354.

Adams, R. (2003). *Social work and empowerment* (3rd ed., pp. 1–27). New York: Palgrave MacMillan.

Alsup, E. (1996). *Liberation psychology: A visionary mandate for humanistic, existential, and transpersonal psychologies.* Retrieved March 2, 2006, from http://www.skaggs-island.org/humanistic/alsup1.html

Austin, S., & Prilleltensky, I. (2001). Diverse origins, common aims: The challenge of critical psychology. *Radical Psychology, 2*(2). Retrieved March 2, 2006, from http://www.radpsynet.org/journal/vol2-2/austin-prilleltensky.html

Ballou, M. (2005). Threats and challenges to feminist therapy. In M. Hill & M. Ballou (Eds.), *The foundation and future of feminist therapy* (pp. 201–210). New York: Haworth Press.

Ballou, M., Matsumoto, A., & Wagner, M. (2002). Toward a feminist ecological theory of human nature: Theory building in the response to the real world dynamics. In M. Ballou & L. Brown (Eds.), *Rethinking mental health and disorder: Feminist perspectives.* New York: Guilford Press.

Bernstein, M. (1997). Celebration and suppression: The strategic use of identity by the lesbian and gay movement. *American Journal of Sociology, 103,* 531–566.

Bernstein, M. (2002). Identity and politics: Toward an understanding of the lesbian and gay movement. *Social Science History, 26*(3), 551–581.

Brabeck, M., & Ting, K. (2000). Introduction [Summary of tenets of feminist theory of psychological practice]. In M. Brabeck (Ed.), *Practicing feminist ethics in psychology.* Washington, DC: American Psychological Association.

Breton, M. (1984). Relating competence: Promotion and empowerment. *Journal of Progressive Human Services, 5*(1), 27–45.

Brown, L. (1994). *Subversive dialogues: Theory in feminist therapy.* New York: Basic Books.

Brown, L., & Ballou, M. (Eds.). (1992). *Personality and psychopathology: Feminist reappraisals.* New York: Guilford Press.

Comas-Diaz, L. (1994). An integrative approach. In L. Comas-Diaz & B. Greene (Eds.), *Women of color* (pp. 287–318). New York: Guilford Press.

Cross, W. (1995). The psychology of Nigrescence: Revising the Cross model. In J. G. Ponterotto, J. Casas, L. Suzuki, & C. Alexander (Eds.), *Handboook of multicultural counseling* (pp. 93–122). Thousand Oaks, CA: Sage.

Edwards, G. (2004). Habermas and social movements: What's "new"? *Sociological Review,* 52(Suppl. 1), 113–130.

Ehrenreich, B., & English, D. (1973). *Witches, midwives and nurses: A history of women healers.* New York: Feminist Press.

Espin, O. (1994). Feminist approaches. In L. Comas-Diaz & B. Greene (Eds.), *Women of color* (pp. 265–286). New York: Guilford Press.

Feminist Therapy Institute. (1999). *Feminist therapy code of ethics.* Retrieved February 12, 2006, from http://www.feminist-therapy-institute.org/ethics.htm

Fraser, N. (2003, February 22–23). *Social justice in globalization.* Introductory talk at the conference Globalizacao: Fatalidade ou Utopia? Coimbra, Portugal.

Giddings, P. (1984). *When and where I enter: The impact of black women on race and sex in America.* New York: Morrow.

Habermas, J. (1981). *The theory of communicative action.* London: Beacon Press.

Hare-Mustin, R. T., & Maracek, J. (1990). *Making a difference: Psychology and the construction of gender.* New Haven, CT: Yale University.

Held, V. (1993). *Feminist morality: Transforming culture, society and politics.* Chicago: University of Chicago Press.

Held, V. (Ed.). (1995). *Justice and care: Essential readings in feminist ethics.* Boulder, CO: Westview Press.

Helms, J. (1995). An update of Helms's white and people of color racial identity models. In J. G. Ponterotto, J. Casas, L. Suzuki, & C. Alexander (Eds.), *Handboook of multicultural counseling* (pp. 181–198). Thousand Oaks, CA: Sage.

Herrick, J. (1995, November 1–3). *Empowerment practice and social change: The place for new social movement theory.* A working draft for the New Social Movement and Community Organizing Conference, University of Washington, Seattle, WA. Retrieved January 10, 2006, from http://www.interweb-tech.com/nsmnet/docs/herrick.htm

hooks, b. (1989). *Talking back: Thinking feminist, thinking black.* Boston: South End Press.

hooks, b., & McKinnon, T. (1996). Sisterhood: Beyond public and private. *Signs, 21*(4), 814–829.

Hutchings, K. (1999). Feminism, universalism, and the ethics of international politics. In V. Jabri & E. O'Gorman (Eds.), *Women, culture and international relations* (pp. 17–38). Boulder, CO: Lynne Reinner.

Jagger, A. (1992). Feminist ethics. In L. Becker & C. Becker (Eds.), *Encyclopedia of ethics* (pp. 363–364). New York: Garland.

Jaggar, A. (1998). Globalizing feminist ethics. *Hypatia, 13*(2), 7–31.

Maracek, J., & Kravetz, D. (1998). Putting politics into practice: Feminist therapy as feminist praxis. *Women & Therapy, 21,* 17–36.

Martin-Baro, I. (1994). *Writing for a liberation psychology.* Cambridge, MA: Harvard University Press.

Monk, G., & Gehart, D. (2003). Sociopolitical activist or conversational partner? Distinguishing the position of the therapist in narrative and collaborative therapies. *Family Process 42*(1), 19–30.

Sparks, E., & Park, A. (2002). The integration of feminism and multiculturalism: Ethical dilemmas at the border. In M. Brabeck (Ed.), *Practicing feminist ethics in psychology*. Washington, DC: American Psychological Association.

Steiner, C., & Wycoff, H. (1975). *Radical psychiatry*. New York: Grove Press.

Tong, R. (2003). Feminist ethics. In E. Zalta (Ed.), *The Stanford encyclopedia of philosophy*. Retrieved February 2, 2006, from http://plato.stanford.edu/archives/win2003/entries/feminism-ethics

Toomey, M. (1992). *Liberation psychology: Calling for revolution not reform*. Retrieved March 2, 2006, from http://www.mtoomey.com/libpsychrev.html

Unger, R. (1998). *Resisting gender: Twenty-five years of feminist psychology*. Thousand Oaks, CA: Sage.

CHAPTER 8

Ethics and Activism:
Application

Claudia Pitts, Liz Margolies, and Elaine Leeder

Psychotherapy, regardless of the orientation of the individual practitioner, is a process that is intended to relieve the suffering of the client. At best, the client will also achieve symptom alleviation, understanding, and a broader repertoire of skills for future problem solving. Most good psychotherapists believe their work is value-free in working with the client toward her or his own stated goals. They also strive to keep themselves personally value-neutral and restrict the intrusion of self into the therapeutic encounter.

In reality, there are limitations to this ideal. Traditional psychotherapies are based on a set of unseen but powerful values, and clients' goals are limited by the futures they are capable of imagining. For both participants in the therapeutic alliance, there is usually an unconscious and unspoken acceptance of the cultural norms, reducing change options to those that fit within society's structures and values as they are perceived now. Worse, traditional psychotherapy limits the focus and change work to that which can be accomplished within a clinical setting, whether it is a 45-minute session in a private practice office or the inpatient mental health unit of the community hospital. The locus of change is placed within the client, or sometimes more broadly, within the family unit.

Feminist therapists understand that real and long-lasting change cannot be accomplished solely in a clinical setting or by focusing solely on the clients themselves. Change must simultaneously take place in the social setting in which the client's difficulties became apparent. In other words, feminist therapy does not end at the walls of the therapy room or at the close of the allotted session time. This crucial aspect of feminist therapy, where change is effected in the environment, is both the most empowering aspect of the treatment and the most controversial and difficult. Feminist therapists believe that engaging in social action on their clients' behalves is not an adjunct to therapy but part and parcel of the treatment program.

Feminist therapists understand that when we walk outside the therapy office, we are entering complicated professional and personal territory. First, few of us have received training in social activism, and it means leaving the setting where we are experts and entering a place where we may have less power and prestige. This can be quite daunting. Second, because social activism has not been considered "therapeutic" work within the insurance and medical models, it is hard for feminist therapists to know how and whether to charge for their time. It may be easier, for example, to bill a family for speaking with a child's teacher than for attending a rally against violence in the schools. Also, after a full and exhausting day seeing clients at the office, it is hard to feel motivated to write a letter to your local newspaper or congressperson. The discomforts and personal challenges pile up, making it feel simpler to minimize the value of work outside the office.

Therapists trained as psychologists or counselors have little professional pressure to involve themselves in work outside the office. Social justice work is not part of the training for either of these professions, nor is it mentioned in either of their ethical codes. Participating in social action may come more easily to therapists who have been trained as social workers. Graduate-level course work addresses the issue, and the ethical code of the National Association of Social Workers (NASW) lists social justice work as one of the profession's core values:

> **VALUE:** Social Justice
> **Ethical Principle:** Social workers challenge social injustice.
> Social workers pursue social change, particularly with and on behalf of vulnerable and oppressed individuals and groups of people. Social workers' social change efforts are focused primarily on issues of poverty, unemployment, discrimination, and other forms of social injustice. These activities seek to promote sensitivity to and knowledge about oppression and cultural and ethnic diversity. Social workers strive to ensure access to needed information, services, and resources; equality of opportunity; and meaningful participation in decision making for all people. (NASW, 1999)

Feminist therapy can be distinguished from social work in several ways. According to the NASW code of ethics, social workers begin their change efforts by addressing unequal access to resources, primarily poverty and unemployment. Feminist therapy begins with a power analysis based on gender. Ideally, in both approaches, the work will ultimately address all forms of oppression and privilege, but the original lens is different. The second primary distinction is that feminist therapists bring their analyses into the clinical setting, revealing and discussing issues of power within the therapeutic relationship. Social activism, then, is part of the therapeutic dialogue and may be engaged in by both the therapist and the client (Feminist Therapy Institute, 1999). There is no single correct use of social activism within feminist therapy. The meaning and type of work outside the office may change with each client and that client's issues and needs. The case examples demonstrate the varied ethical uses of social activism.

SCOTT

Scott, the 9-year-old Caucasian boy referred by his school because of his social difficulties, would most likely be referred to a community mental health clinic or practitioner covered by his family's insurance plan. His working parents could not have easily afforded a private practitioner outside of the network, should there be any available in the small Midwestern town where he lives. Upon intake with a qualified social worker or psychologist, the rich story of Scott and his relationship with his world would be entered into his case record. It would be clear that his major difficulty is with his social environment. Scott's relationship with his parents is generally positive and supportive. His grades, though not exceptional, are not cause for alarm. Scott appears to be aware that his body and gender expression make him a target for teasing by other boys. Sometimes his frustration and hurt explode in anger. Intervening at this point in his life may ensure that his grades do not deteriorate, his behavioral problems do not lead to suspension, and his anger does not turn to depression or rage.

Regardless of the type of therapist, Scott's therapy would focus on alleviating his current level of suffering. The particular training of his therapist would determine the method used, but traditional therapy consistently places the locus of change within the client and, perhaps more broadly, within his nuclear family. If Scott were assigned a traditional therapist, the focus might be a combination of helping him to "fit in" and increasing his self-esteem, which would result from the changes he might make in his own behavior and adjustment. If he were assigned a behavioral therapist, the focus might emphasize developing coping skills, learning to "not take the teasing personally" and encouraging "appropriate" interactions with male peers. He may be guided to lose weight, become more physical, and cut his hair, all of which would make him less of a target to his peers and, therefore, less angry, at least outwardly. The success of this treatment would be measured by less "acting out" behavior at school. If Scott were assigned a more psychodynamic psychotherapist, the treatment might examine the underlying issues behind the aggressive and nonconforming behaviors, focusing first on Scott's rejection of masculinity. Together, the clinician and Scott would uncover his family dynamics and investigate whether Scott's identification with or rejection of his father is a root cause. If a family therapist were brought in for adjunctive treatment, she might look across the generations at the history of "feminine" men in Scott's family, their subsequent rejection from their primary social settings (church and school), and the anger that ensued.

These techniques and assumptions might help to relieve some of Scott's distress. He would certainly become more clear about having a "choice" about how to dress and behave, as well as understand the consequences of his appearance and behavior. In this way, the work could be considered empowering. But the power to choose to "fit in" (or not) is a limited power indeed. Scott's symptoms and distress would best be addressed by a treatment (and value system) that begins by supporting him in both discovering and expressing his authentic self, helping him question the "health" of the school environment, and encouraging him to form connections with other youth who either share or respect his gender expression. The most important and enduring changes for Scott would come out of the feminist therapy work, that takes place outside of the office.

An open and feminist ear hears one of the most striking dynamics in this case: Scott does not express unhappiness with himself. Other than feeling clumsy, he has not stated a desire to be different. His parents, the school staff, his peers, and, very likely, his church are the ones who see Scott as having a problem with his gender identity. Scott seems relatively comfortable with his dress and choice of play. He "acts out" only in response to harassment. Although at 9 years old, Scott would express it more simply, he appears to be quite aware of the hegemony of the cultural norm of masculinity. In fact, his actions in defense of self seem quite sensible, if neither effective nor appropriate.

Feminist therapists see the flaw in placing the "burden of change upon the individual as the one who needs to change, not upon the system that is represented as stable and normative" (Roffman, early version of Chapter 7, this volume). However, there may be aspects of himself that Scott wishes to change, and a feminist therapist would offer him the opportunity to voice his own desires about it. He needs an opportunity to think about how, if at all, he would like to alter his behavior, his gender expression (more masculine *or* more feminine), his position within his family, his relationship with other boys, and his role in the school. It is important that these changes be based not on a sense of his own inadequacy or pathology, but on a powerful belief that change is possible and will create a more satisfying life for him.

The most distinctive aspect of treatment with a feminist therapist would be working with Scott to explore what things *in his world* might be alterable. The challenge here is not to change Scott, but rather to work on changing the system. According to Fraser (2003), as quoted in Roffman (Chapter 7, this volume), "The work of feminist therapy is directed toward changing the social arrangements that perpetuate inequities as well as the work of creating cultural systems that promote and encourage self esteem and respect within and for individuals." Scott can be seen as an "expert" in his own care, making the decisions about where he would like to see change in his environment. Change can be worked on simultaneously within his family, his school, and his community. To accomplish these changes, his therapist must educate herself about gender nonconformity and become familiar with the community organizations and social justice groups in her area that are working on the issues. It is the feminist therapist's responsibility to engage with the issues outside the therapy room, in the greater society, and to help those with whom she works to do the same.

A feminist therapist may also work with Scott's parents, empowering them to act as advocates for their son in the school system and community, rather than to lovingly manipulate Scott into tolerability. His parents can be helped to see that, within their home, Scott does not demonstrate anger and dysfunction. They have created an affectionate and emotionally expressive family setting by being "tolerant of who he is," allowing Scott to play with dolls without censure. In this warm environment, he is noted to be a particularly "loving" child. The setting determines how Scott is perceived and, therefore, how he behaves. At home, he is a "gentle man." At school, the same behaviors get him rejected and called a "girlie-girl." The parents can be helped to see that the best way to protect their child's self-esteem is to work to make the school environment better match the tolerance Scott receives at home. His mother can be reminded that she is a manager at work and that this, at one time, would not have been acceptable for a woman. Parallels can be drawn to how society had to change for her to be able to express this part of herself. This is also true for Scott's father. His role as an "involved dad" was one that required societal change in order to be seen as viable.

An activist approach, for the therapist, might entail working with the school to address issues of gender conformity, offering a workshop, training staff, or investigating how many other students (male and female) may be experiencing similar problems. Some of the students may appear gender-conforming but experience great stress over the pressure to conform. The therapist does not work alone. Using her access to community groups working on this issue increases her resources and builds connections. The greater the size and diversity of the group that approaches the school, the greater the influence the group can have. Many groups have prepared curricula for schools around gender expression and safety. One such group may have colleagues within Scott's school that can facilitate the process of instituting a staff training or program for students. It might also be useful to connect Scott with similar kids through a group in the community or to help organize such a group at his school.

To summarize, a feminist approach to Scott's situation recognizes that it is not the role of the therapist to protect or rescue Scott from "the world" and its negative views of him, but rather to empower him and his family to be change agents in the creation of a world where Scott finds himself able to be his "best self" without fear of judgment or rejection.

ANNA AND SERGEI

A traditional therapist might approach the case of Anna and Sergei, recent immigrants, with a focus on improving their adjustment to their current situation. It makes sense to believe that if they were better able to manage the stressors accompanying their immigration and son Sasha's illness, it might make them more able to seek employment, access the health care system, improve their English, and create a social support network in their neighborhood.

Although any therapist would certainly see the economic pressures on this family as substantive and central to their problems, it is the understanding of these issues in a larger context, beginning with a focus on gender, that differentiates the feminist and traditional viewpoints. A feminist analysis would address the nature and social value of Anna's work. Even before they came to this country, Anna's work was not considered "career track," whereas Sergei's work, as an apprentice, was. In the United States, only his job offered medical benefits, reinforcing the belief that it is the man's responsibility to provide the main income and benefits for his family and that women's work, especially if she is not college-educated, is less valuable and deserves lower pay and no benefits.

Feminist therapists understand the interconnectedness of all forms of oppression. Anna and Sergei's difficulties are not uniquely their own but are connected to larger issues of immigration, health care, and unemployment. Again, as with Scott, the feminist therapist must move beyond the office walls and educate herself about these issues. Simultaneously, she would work to connect Sergei and Anna to existing immigrant rights groups or help them begin to informally create their own. Of course, it is incumbent upon the therapist not to "force" a political agenda on the client or overburden an already overwhelmed family, but rather to help them see their difficulties as having a social and political basis, not just as an expression of their personal failings. This perspective lifts the added burden of shame and allows them to see their issues as shared, current, and remediable. In this aspect of the work, feminist therapists, not denying their value base, make clear the values present in their work and allow those with whom they work to accept or reject them as they choose. When the values underlying therapy are unseen or unacknowledged, they can be experienced as critical judgments and serve to unwittingly silence the clients.

If Sergei and Anna choose to work for change within society, rather than focusing solely on themselves and their immediate family, they will feel empowered to create change in themselves, their community, and perhaps society as a whole. At a minimum, connecting with others in their neighborhood to work for change will begin the formation of a social support network, opening them up to job possibilities and potential babysitters, as well as the chance to make a difference and make friends. In other words, working on social change facilitates individual change.

ABBY

Abby, the sexual abuse survivor, presents a case in which gender politics are at the forefront. Child sexual abuse continues to be a crime mostly committed by men against girls, and yet society continues to question the innocence of the female victims. This stance isolates girls from each other and daughters from their mothers. Girls carry the shame of the crime within themselves and too often engage in behaviors that are self-destructive. Abby's decision to not tell anyone of her abuse caused her problems above and beyond the damage of the abuse itself.

Most traditional therapists would interpret Abby's anxiety, alcohol use, and chronic benzodiazepine use to be a result of her sexual assault. Most therapists would look at ways for Abby to reduce her anxiety so as not to require the continued use of anxiolytics. Depending on the therapist's orientation and training, Abby might be trained in relaxation exercises and ways to cope in potentially difficult situations. She might be referred to a 12-step program to help her eliminate her dependence on medication. She would be encouraged to improve her self-esteem and boundaries in order to feel a sense of control in her life.

A feminist therapist might well do some or all of theses things, but would also work at helping Abby to reduce her level of distress. However, a therapy that keeps her solely focused on her own behavior, difficulties, and addictions would be limited in its effectiveness. As stated previously, one of the worst aspects of the crime of childhood sexual abuse is the isolation it creates. Abby's treatment must include methods of connecting her to other people, especially her mother and other women who have also internalized the shame of sexual abuse. Ideally, she would come to understand her particular story within the larger history of African American women and sexual control. It is incumbent on Abby's therapist to understand this history as well and to do whatever she can to make changes in their community. Understanding how abuse and its secrecy is harming girls everywhere, the therapist may want to make sure that there are programs at the local schools to help adults recognize when girls may be being sexually abused at home. She may offer to train teachers and staff. This kind of social activism not only would be helpful to Abby but also would contribute to the self-care of the therapist. Working year after year with the adult scars from childhood victimization can be debilitating or disheartening for a therapist. As with Abby herself, being part of the change effort is empowering for all.

CONCLUSION

Feminist therapy is more than a method of doing therapy; it is a movement for social change that works at challenging the dominant paradigms of our time, particularly as they relate to gender. Feminist therapists are continually working to become more aware of race, class, and ethnicity and other dimensions of oppression; we work toward social justice and challenge the systems of institutionalized inequity. In these three cases, it has been shown that therapists must be conscious of power inequities in the classroom, at home, in the therapeutic hour, and in society. A feminist therapist strives to be an activist, a role model, a challenger of the status quo, and an "inside agitator," lobbying for social justice while still working with clients to relieve the stresses that postmodern society presents. Feminist therapy is still relevant in the twenty-first century because the systems of power and privilege remain. We, and our clients, need to challenge these systems from both inside and outside the system and the office. We invite the reader to join us in those challenges.

REFERENCES

Feminist Therapy Institute. (1995). Feminist therapy code of ethics. In E. Rave & E. Larsen (Eds.), *Ethical decision making in therapy: Feminist perspectives*. New York: Guilford Press.

National Association of Social Workers. (1999). *Code of ethics for social workers*. Washington, DC: NASW Press.

CHAPTER 9

Putting It All Together: *Theory*

Marcia Hill and Jae Y. Jeong

BACKGROUND

Thus far, we have looked at the context of therapy: the political and sociocultural settings in which the practice of therapy occurs. We have considered the person of the client, investigating how the client's characteristics and identity will affect that person's therapy. We have examined the practice of therapy itself, in terms of both a multifaceted approach to understanding human pain and feminist adaptations of various ways to intervene with that pain. And we have looked at ethics and activism as an integral part of how we understand and enact therapy. Now we will integrate all of these elements into a feminist conceptualization of psychotherapy.

Feminist therapy is a complex and sophisticated endeavor. The traditional model (Figure 9.1), and especially the insurance-driven model of psychotherapy, looks as follows:

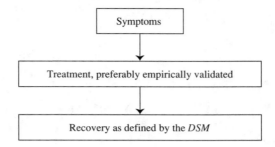

In a feminist model of psychotherapy, possible biological or intrapsychic contributors to distress are only a partial beginning. The feminist model looks more like this:

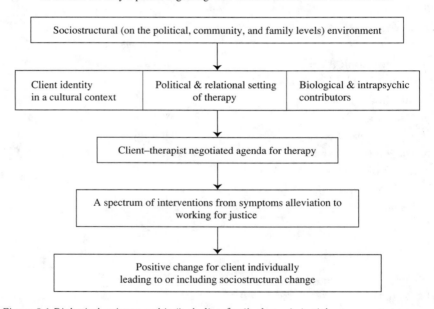

Figure 9.1 Biological or intrapsychic (including family dynamics) etiology.

More specifically, the feminist therapist recognizes that injury is not random, but is powerfully influenced by bias and by unequal distribution of resources. Many injuries are an expression of that inequality, and most injuries have at least a component of it. In such a context, the client's position in the culture becomes of paramount importance in understanding not only the nature and meaning of the client's experience, but also the nature and meaning of the client's injuries. Further, therapy occurs not in a vacuum, but in a political climate that implies corporate ownership of therapy (Ballou & Hill, Chapter 1, this volume) and that sees therapy as something "done to" the client with the client's role limited to cooperation or failure to cooperate and defines injury as intrapsychic or biological disorder. Given these factors, a client's recovery is limited because the client continues to live in a cultural context that is destructive in a variety of ways. (Gentile, Kisber, Suvak, & West discuss this in more detail in Chapter 5 of this volume.) Working for justice thus becomes the ultimate therapeutic act.

The role of the therapist is to work collaboratively with the client in understanding and responding to the client's difficulties, keeping in mind that much of what is helpful is a stance that communicates client ownership of the therapy and an understanding of human pain that recognizes a picture much larger than the situation of the individual client. As Ballou and Hill describe in Chapter 1 of this volume, recognizing the larger sociostructural context of the client's difficulties and incorporating that understanding into the therapy is central to a feminist therapeutic stance. Thus, the feminist therapist negotiates both the therapy goals and its process with the client. Feminist therapy is not a technique, but a way of thinking about therapy, about the etiology of problems, about responses to pain or injury, and about how to help. The practice of feminist therapy thus not only conceptualizes psychotherapy politically, but also *enacts* that conceptualization. We look at this in more detail as this chapter continues.

A WAY TO THINK ABOUT THERAPY

All aspects of how one interacts with a client convey something about who is in charge (Leupnitz, 1988). Does the therapist make the diagnosis, or does she discuss it with the client? Does the therapist respond behind the scenes to insurance company requirements for information, or is the client actively involved in choosing how to respond to these requirements? What does the office and waiting room convey about what kinds of clients are expected or welcome (Weiner, 1998)? The feminist therapist thinks about the setting and business aspects of therapy as potential contributors to either the status quo or change.

In addition, much of what makes therapy feminist is the articulation of the hidden. It is not only the understanding of the effects of bias and injustice that make for feminist therapy, but also the naming of these components. Naming the cultural contributors to abuse, body image discomfort, isolation, economic insecurity, self-esteem problems, and the like is a powerful antidote to shame. In addition, recognizing the sociocultural elements of any difficulty opens the door to addressing those factors directly, if there are elements that the client can influence, while not presuming that the client has personal control over the entirety of her situation. Recognizing the social construction of dominance, as described by Roffman (Chapter 7, this volume), is central to feminist therapy.

A WAY TO THINK ABOUT THE ETIOLOGY OF PROBLEMS

Injustice and Hate Crimes

What are the sources of emotional distress? You will notice that we are not talking about "behavior" here, which is merely one way that distress can be manifested. Many times a person's behavior looks fine to observers, while the individual's internal experience is causing significant suffering. Pain is experienced and expressed in multiple ways.

Much pain is caused by injustice in one form or another. In the largest sense, the injustices of racism, sexism, and so forth cause much human suffering, manifest through multiple avenues. What therapist has not tried to help heterosexual couples who are struggling with the difficulties caused by the household division of labor? Sexist assumptions on the part of both women and men continue to create difficulties for both sexes. This manifests both practically and internally. Thus, for example, on the practical or external level, both sexes may assume that women have primary administrative responsibility for household labor and child care, with men "helping." Less overtly, both sexes may feel that a male who earns less than his female partner is less masculine. These kinds of examples are old news but continue to be virtually universal today. Changes to some of the structural barriers to gender equality, such as parental leave for both sexes and increased representation of women in some kinds of jobs, have left problems in this less public area relatively untouched.

Similarly, statistics continue to show most people of color being paid less than white people, having poorer medical care than whites, and so forth, with disparities depending on the particular group and the nature of the racialized injustice (Bound, Waidmann, Schoenbaum, & Bingenheimer, 2003; De Leon, Barnes, Bienias, Skarupski, & Evans, 2005; Epstein, 2004; Johnson, Roter, Powe, & Cooper, 2004; Woolf, Johnson, Fryer, Rust, & Satcher, 2004). Research indicates that fat people earn less than their thinner counterparts (Brown & Rothblum, 1989). Barriers not only to employment, but also to full participation in civic life, are an ongoing challenge to people with disabilities (Federici et al., 2005; Melville et al., 2006; Olkin, 1999; Piggott, Sapey, & Wilenius, 2005). Limited access to transportation, interpreter services, adaptive technology, and personal care assistance is a stressor faced by those with disabilities that is no more or less than the stress of injustice made manifest.

Many times the effect of injustice is internal, but no less substantial for being experienced psychologically. Barrett and Ballou (Chapter 3, this volume) examine the complexities of identity and the struggles and risks that can result from either dominant or nondominant identities. Consider an adolescent girl whose developing sexual pull is toward other girls. If she comes of age in a community where gay and lesbian people are invisible, or worse, openly scorned, she will likely suffer as a result. Imagine the impoverished Hispanic youth whose school is inadequate, whose community lacks resources, and who is regularly looked down on by others when he ventures out of his neighborhood. This is not a specific trauma in the same way that violence is, but it is traumatic nonetheless (Root, 1996), and this child will almost certainly show the effects of living in the injurious context of racism and poverty. Consider the African American man who sees fear in the eyes of white people as he walks downtown. Think of the woman in a wheelchair who feels invisible because no one meets her gaze. Imagine a man of 60 who cannot find a job and wonders how much of that is a simple unwillingness to hire a person of his age. Contemplate the life choices available to a young person of either gender who grows up in poverty. None of these phenomena are particularly visible, or even in many cases discrete, events, yet they cause pain as surely as a more direct injury. In many cases, the effect may be worse than that of a specific trauma, because of the chronicity of the experience and because its invisibility may lead the individual to see it as a personal failing rather than an expression of injustice. The feminist therapist recognizes a continuum of violence (Brown, 2004; Caplan, 1992; Sharma, 2001), with all acts of oppression being a form of violence as surely as is assault. Violence is shockingly common, but the hate crimes of poverty, racism, homophobia, and the like are more common still.

Many—perhaps most—forms of interpersonal violence are also a result of injustice. Most obvious are what are legally considered "hate crimes," that is, a crime committed against someone because of her or his membership in a particular group. Violence against gay men is a common example, with the perpetrators often making clear statements indicating that the victims were targeted specifically because of their sexual orientation. However, violence against women might frequently also fall into the category of hate crimes. Most rape is an example of this (Balsam, 2003; Brownmiller, 1975; McPhail & DiNitto, 2005; Renzetti & Bergen, 2005). Less directly, poverty, complicated by the injuries of racism and other forms of injustice, creates settings that invites higher crime rates. The violence thus generated is certainly a form of violence resulting from injustice, even if the connection is mediated by other variables such as despair, lower police protection, or drug and alcohol abuse. Domestic violence presents a somewhat different picture. In this case, women may not be targeted specifically because of gender. However, male-perpetrated domestic violence is commonly one expression of male entitlement and control, leading us back to gendered injustice as a primary causal element (Dutton, 1998; Hyden, 2005). The same is true with childhood sexual abuse, in which most perpetrators are male (Hanson, Gizzarelli, & Scott, 1994; Smallbone & Wortley, 2004). In that case, entitlement may be intertwined with a kind of ownership mentality regarding children: a combination of the effects of age-related and gender-related injustice (Marziano, Ward, Beech, & Pattison, 2006).

In summary, many clients in psychotherapists' offices are the casualties of injustice. They are traumatized by childhood sexual abuse, by rape, by sexual harassment, and by domestic terrorism. They suffer from the effects of overt discrimination and an apportioning of resources that leaves many without necessities such as medical care, or an education appropriate to their talents, or even basic safety. And most insidiously, they are affected by the chronic low-level injuries of being seen by others as "less than" in some way.

Let us recognize also that injustice injures those who are privileged as well as those oppressed by it. Guilt, whether conscious or not, is a common outcome. Often those with greater privilege are constrained by that very privilege, with certain life choices being unavailable or disparaged. In addition, the culture of privilege, whether it be a consequence of gender, race, wealth, or any other status, encourages complicity with a system that entitles some at the expense of others. The injuries of the disadvantaged are founded on the cooperation of those who are advantaged. Surely cooperation with injustice takes its toll even on the advantaged. And all of us, on whatever point in each spectrum of privilege, are impoverished by every fellow human who is prevented from making the contribution that is hers or his alone to make.

Circumstance

Sometimes the distress that brings people to seek help is simply the result of circumstance. Some people are predisposed to a sunny disposition, others to depression. Some people, through genetics or good fortune, are physically vigorous; others experience debilitating challenges to health or physical functioning. That said, virtually all kinds of difficulties are made easier for those with greater resources. Money buys better medical care, for example, particularly in the United States. Those who do not have added life stressors such as dealing with a disability or being an immigrant may be better able to cope with the aftermath of a car accident. And some injustices, with poverty and the complex intertwining of poverty and racism being the most obvious examples, make one far more likely to be hard hit by some kinds of "bad luck," such as natural disasters. However, to some extent, illness, accidents, natural disasters, loss, and other painful experiences are democratic: no one escapes at least some of these life events.

Other effects of happenstance are more subtle: Is the person physically attractive and coordinated? Is she more outgoing or shy? Does he tend to put on weight? Yet even these factors are influenced by cultural biases that favor coordination over, say, empathy; extroversion over introversion; thinness over bulk.

The task of the therapist in these cases is to untangle the effects of the event itself from the complications of injustices that might make a person more vulnerable or less able to respond effectively. Being in a car accident might simply be a result of bad luck. Being unable to afford a reliable car in the first place or having inadequate insurance because of poverty is a consequence of injustice. One kind of suffering might be unavoidable; the other is not.

The Map of the Self

There is a place in feminist therapy, as in all therapy, for recognizing an intrapsychic etiology of problems. Pain is the result not only of injustice and circumstance, but also of the limitations that result from an individual's assumptions about who she is and about the nature of human relationships. This is the traditional model of psychology: failures in parenting or mismatches between the caregiver and the child can result in injuries and limitations. In addition, there are many other situations (sibling relationships, school experiences, community support or difficulties) that influence the developing child's sense of who she is and what she can expect from relationships. A boy whose caregivers are unresponsive, because of alcoholism, for example, may develop into an adult whose self-esteem comes from rescuing others and who believes that he cannot get his needs met in relationships. This can be thought of as a flawed or limited "map" of the self and of relationships, a template that does not include the enormous possibilities available in the world and instead narrows to assumptions that mirror the circumstances of the family. Even something as typically private to a family as alcoholism, however, occurs in a community context, and with adequate community resources and intervention, the effects for this child of growing up in such a family might have been mitigated.

Differences between a child and caregiver that result in chronic misunderstanding are another way that people form limiting and hurtful maps of self and relationships. A child whose talents are mechanical can easily feel disparaged and unappreciated if she grows up in a family that values books and language instead. In this case, the girl might well feel ashamed and inadequate, with an inclination toward relationships with individuals who look down on her in the way that she finds familiar.

In addition, as any parent can tell you, each child arrives with her or his own temperament, strengths, and vulnerabilities. One person may be more inclined to anxiety, another to moodiness. One may have an organized and logical mind; another may be a creative and divergent thinker. These kinds of innate characteristics may sometimes bring people to the attention of therapists if the characteristics are problematic in the person's life context (e.g., a manager whose tendency toward perfectionism leads him to relational difficulties in the workplace) or if they are salient enough to cause problems. An example of the latter would be someone whose vulnerability to depression is severe enough to require intervention. We should remember, too, that some kinds of strengths, particularly those associated with school success and congruent with the child's gender and community expectations, are rewarded, whereas others may be ignored or actively disparaged.

However, it is important for therapists to recognize, as Barrett and Ballou (Chapter 3, this volume) argue, that no individual has a unitary "self." Each person has many identities or expressions of identity that vary depending on the situation. The self is shaped in the context of the person's culture (both social and political), community, and family. It will also be shaped in the context of the therapy climate and relationship. In addition, therapy occurs during a particular point in history and in a specific geographic location. These kinds of macro-factors can be so taken for granted that they become invisible, yet they can be significant influences on the assumptions, resources, and limitations of both therapist and client (Barrett & Ballou, this volume).

A WAY TO THINK ABOUT RESPONSES TO PAIN

Rare is the therapist who believes that the same kind of intervention is appropriate with every problem. Therapists change what they do depending on the style of the individual client and on the nature of the client's difficulty. But in the same way that different problems may require different forms of help, one must look at the etiology of the problem and consider that when crafting a way to help. Thus, a client who is anxious simply because it is her nature will need a different approach from someone who is anxious because he was the victim of a hate crime. Both may need to develop anxiety-management skills, but beyond that, the therapist's approach will differ. Here we focus not on technique, but on how to conceptualize an approach to helping that takes into account the etiology of the problem. Notice how this conceptualization is in itself political. Feminist therapy begins its enactment of its politics with understanding of nature of the problem and by offering solutions that are in themselves politicized.

Isolation and Shame Versus Solidarity and Action

People who have been victimized, either by violence or by the subtler trauma of oppression, often feel shame and isolation (Herman, 1992). "Blaming the victim" is a common response to those who have experienced violence (Henning & Holdford, 2006) and is a way that others maintain an illusion of invulnerability. In addition, those victimized may feel shame either from internalized oppression (Cohen, 2005) or as a way to maintain the illusion that they had the power to prevent the violence. Isolation is a natural outcome of shame. People who are victimized commonly presume that others will see or respond to them as they do to themselves. Thus, they may withdraw from intimacy out of a wish to avoid being seen as "bad," damaged, at fault, or objects of pity. Clients with a history of abuse or other victimization often report to therapists that they have told few others about the experience.

A powerful antidote to shame and isolation is to tell of one's injury, particularly in the company of others who have had similar experiences (Breton & Nosko, 2005; Kees & Leech, 2004; Kreidler & England, 1990). It is hard for a client to maintain self-blame when she hears the stories of other people, people who have been injured in ways similar to her and who clearly did not "ask for" or deserve that injury. For example, a client who sits in a room with several other women who have experienced domestic terrorism will be much less likely to believe that her experience is unique or somehow the result of her personal failings. As Gentile, Kisber, Suvak, and West (Chapter 5, this volume) describe, simply examining one's assumptions about the causes of injury can be helpful. In the context of shared injury, people can come to see that "the personal is political," that is, that their individual experiences are part of a larger pattern that is the outgrowth of forces other than their specific situations.

This is also true for those injuries that are the outcome of the more insidious forms of violence: racism, fat oppression, homophobia, and other forms of identity- or status-based bias. Thus, a deaf client who feels frustrated, alone, and weary of fighting for appropriate accommodations needs not only support from his therapist but also solidarity with other deaf people. Women, people of color, and gay and lesbian people have generally made good strides in recognizing the need for the company of others like themselves, both for support and as a way to organize for change. But people affected by bias based on age, size, disability, immigrant status, and class have often been less likely to organize. Roffman (Chapter 7, this volume) notes particularly our limited integration of a class analysis into therapy. Therapy is only a small component of a helpful response to these kinds of insidious traumas, and locating resources and encouraging the client to participate in groups of like others, whether for socialization or to organize for change, is an important part of healing.

Individual Responsibility Versus Community and Social Policy Support

When it comes to pain that is the result of circumstance or events such as loss, accidents, illness, natural disasters, and the like, few people have all the resources they need for a full and adequate response. The feminist therapist recognizes that the difficulties of these kinds of injuries are often compounded by social policy that limits resources available to people in need. Resources are frequently even more meager in communities of color or in poor communities. Thus, the presumption that people can and should be personally responsible for their recovery from tragedy ignores the reality that decisions made at the national or state level about resources such as medical care and disaster assistance will greatly affect each person's ability to recover. In addition, as mentioned previously, communities with fewer resources are often hardest hit by what appears to be bad luck or circumstance. A lifelong history of inadequate medical care may result in a higher rate of life-threatening illness in some communities, for example. Thus we see higher rates of some illnesses (Farmer, 2005) and shorter life expectancies (Mueller, Ortega, Parker, Patil, & Askenazi, 1999) among those people who have not only the fewest personal resources but also the fewest community resources.

Medical-Model Pathologizing Versus Collaborative Problem Solving

In looking at kinds of distress that originate primarily in problems with one's map of the world or of the self, the therapist's conceptualization and responses can either subtly add to the problem or ease it. Much of how psychotherapy is structured, particularly in terms of third-party reimbursement, presumes a medical model that describes the client as deficient in some way and the therapist as doing something "to" the client to effect change. Ballou and Hill (Chapter 1, this volume) examine particularly the ways that corporate control of therapy has exacerbated this stance. The most obvious example of this is the requirement for a diagnosis—and, for that matter, the system of diagnoses itself. Required "treatment plans," discussions (either written or verbal) between insurance company representatives and therapists, and some kinds of record-keeping requirements all contribute to a picture that implies a passive client and a therapist in charge of treating that client.

Much of the work in feminist therapy theory has addressed this presumption and described the harm that it does (Ballou, 1995; Brown & Ballou, 1992; Enns, 1992; Kaschak, 1992; Rawlings & Carter, 1977). In addition, a great deal has been written about how to work differently with clients—that is, the importance of creating a collaborative relationship and of adapting therapy practice, from diagnosis to intervention, in a way that is feminist (Brown, 1990; Brown & Ballou, 1992; Enns; Hill, 2004; Hill & Ballou, 1998; Kaschak, 1992; Leupnitz, 1988). To summarize this writing, working with clients in a way that is respectful and collaborative not only tends to create better solutions because it makes good use of the client's expertise about herself, but also avoids the harm that can be a result of working from a stance that can perpetuate injury by treating the client in a way that replicates a cultural misuse of power.

A WAY TO THINK ABOUT HELPING

Feminist therapy runs the gamut from symptom alleviation to working for justice. However, all forms of symptom alleviation, as discussed by Tabol and Walker in Chapter 6 of this volume, will be informed by an awareness of the feminist principles of valuing the experience of the client and attention to power in the therapeutic relationship (Hill & Ballou, 1998). Thus, there is no technique separate from an awareness of political context. Further, because much of what brings people to therapy would best be described as the personal manifestation of sociostructural injustices (Hill & Ballou), working for justice is central to the therapeutic endeavor and is entwined with any other ways in which the therapist responds to the client's distress. Roffman (Chapter 7, this volume) cautions against an androcentric model that presumes that public political action is the only legitimate form of activism. She indicates that the act of linking the structures of social control with the experiences of the individual might fall under a broader definition of activism. This, in fact, is a primary goal of feminist therapy. The feminist principles of using an integrated analysis of oppression and recognizing that the ultimate goal of feminist therapy is social change are at work here (Ballou & Hill, Chapter 1).

Because feminist therapy is a process of collaboration with the client at many levels, the therapist will focus much attention on the client's strengths. When working together toward a goal, it is only sensible to make full use of the resources available in both (or all) people involved. Gentile et al. (Chapter 5, this volume) describe in more detail the centrality of collaboration in feminist therapy. Choices about how to proceed are guided by the therapist's knowledge and experience of what tends to work in a given situation and the client's knowledge and experience about what she has found or is finding helpful. In all cases, those choices will heavily favor drawing on the client's personal resources, such as having a logical mind, a good support system, skill in comforting herself, a solid spiritual grounding, a well-honed intuitive ability, and the like. Focus on the client's unique ways of shaping and contributing to the outcome that she wants is central to collaboration.

CONCLUDING COMMENTS

We see, then, that the role of the therapist is to think on many levels simultaneously. The political context of therapy; the sociostructural contributors to the problem; and the person of the client on the individual, relational, and cultural levels will inform each choice that the therapist makes in understanding a problem and in finding a way to help. As discussed previously (Barrett & Ballou, Chapter 3), no client can be understood separate from her environment. Similarly, no client difficulty can be fully comprehended without an appreciation of the cultural context of that problem. No therapy can be conducted without recognition that therapy occurs in a specific political context. And no therapy can be considered complete without an ongoing reference to the principles of justice.

REFERENCES

Ballou, M. (1995). Naming the issue. In E. J. Rave & C. C. Larsen (Eds.), *Ethical decision-making in therapy: Feminist perspectives* (pp. 42–56). New York: Guilford Press.

Balsam, K. F. (2003). Traumatic victimization in the lives of lesbian and bisexual women: A contextual approach. *Journal of Lesbian Studies, 7*(1), 1–14.

Bound, J., Waidmann, T., Schoenbaum, M., & Bingenheimer, J. B. (2003). The labor market consequences of race differences in health. *Milbank Quarterly, 81*(3), 441–473.

Breton, M., & Nosko, A. (2005). Group work with women who have experienced abuse. In G. L. Greif & P. H. Ephross (Eds.), *Group work with populations at risk* (2nd ed., pp. 212–225). New York: Oxford University Press.

Brown, L. (1990). The meaning of a multicultural perspective for theory-building in feminist therapy. In L. Brown & M. Root (Eds.), *Diversity and complexity in feminist therapy* (pp. 1–21). New York: Haworth Press.

Brown, L. (2004). Feminist paradigms of trauma treatment. *Psychotherapy: Theory, Research, Practice, Training, 41*(4), 464–471.

Brown, L., & Ballou, M. (Eds.). (1992). *Personality and psychopathology: Feminist reappraisals*. New York: Guilford Press.

Brown, L., & Rothblum, E. (Eds.). (1989). *Fat oppression and psychotherapy: A feminist perspective*. New York: Haworth Press.

Brownmiller, S. (1975). *Against our will: Men, women, and rape*. New York: Simon & Schuster.

Caplan, P. J. (1992). Driving us crazy: How oppression damages women's mental health and what we can do about it. *Women & Therapy, 12*(3), 5–28.

Cohen, O. (2005). How do we recover? An analysis of psychiatric survivor oral histories. *Journal of Humanistic Psychology, 45*(3), 333–354.

de Leon, C. F., Barnes, L. L., Bienias, J. L., Skarupski, K. A., & Evans, D. A. (2005). Racial disparities in disability: Recent evidence from self-reported and performance-based disability measures in a population-based study of older adults. *Journals of Gerontology: Series B: Psychological Sciences and Social Sciences, 60B*(5), S263–S271.

Dutton, D. G. (1998). *The abusive personality: Violence and control in intimate relationships*. New York: Guilford Press.

Enns, C. (1992). Toward integrating feminist psychotherapy and feminist philosophy. *Professional Psychology: Research and Practice, 23*(6), 453–466.

Epstein, A. (2004). Health care in America—Still too separate, not yet equal. *New England Journal of Medicine, 351*(6), 603–605.

Farmer, M. (2005). Are racial disparities in health conditional on socioeconomic status? *Social Science & Medicine, 60*(1), 191–204.

Federici, S., Micangeli, A., Ruspantini, I., Borgianni, S., Corradi, F., Pasqualotto, E., et al. (2005). Checking an integrated model of web accessibility and usability evaluation for disabled people. *Disability and Rehabilitation: An International Multidisciplinary Journal, 27*(13), 781–790.

Hanson, R. K., Gizzarelli, R., & Scott, H. (1994). The attitudes of incest offenders: Sexual entitlement and acceptance of sex with children. *Criminal Justice and Behavior, 21*(2), 187–202.

Henning, K., & Holdford, R. (2006). Minimization, denial, and victim blaming by batterers: How much does the truth matter? *Criminal Justice and Behavior, 33*(1), 110–130.

Herman, J. (1992). *Trauma and recovery*. New York: Basic Books.

Hill, M. (2004). *Diary of a country therapist*. New York: Haworth Press.

Hill, M., & Ballou, M. (1998). Making therapy feminist: A practice survey. In M. Hill (Ed.), *Feminist therapy as a political act* (pp. 1–16). New York: Haworth Press.

Hyden, M. (2005). "I must have been an idiot to let it go on": Agency and positioning in battered women's narratives of leaving. *Feminism & Psychology, 15*(2), 169–188.

Johnson, R. L., Roter, D., Powe, N. R., & Cooper, L. A. (2004). Patient race/ethnicity and quality of patient-physician communication during medical visits. *American Journal of Public Health, 94*(12), 2084–2090.

Kaschak, E. (1992). *Engendered lives: A new psychology of women's experience.* New York: Basic Books.

Kees, N., & Leech, N. (2004). Practice trends in women's groups: An inclusive view. In J. L. DeLucia-Waack, D. A. Gerrity, C. R. Kalodner, & M. T. Root (Eds.), *Handbook of group counseling and psychotherapy* (pp. 445–455). Thousand Oaks, CA: Sage.

Kreidler, M. C., & England, D. B. (1990). Empowerment through group support: Adult women who are survivors of incest. *Journal of Family Violence, 5*(1), 35–42.

Leupnitz, D. A. (1988). *The family interpreted.* New York: Basic Books.

Marziano, V., Ward, T., Beech, A. R., & Pattison, P. (2006). Identification of five fundamental implicit theories underlying cognitive distortions in child abusers: A preliminary study. *Psychology, Crime & Law, 12*(1), 97–105.

McPhail, B. A., & DiNitto, D. M. (2005). Prosecutorial perspectives on gender-bias hate crimes. *Violence Against Women, 11*(9), 1162–1185.

Melville, C. A., Cooper, S. A., Morrison, J., Finlayson, J., Allan, L., Robinson, N., et al. (2006). The outcomes of an intervention study to reduce the barriers experienced by people with intellectual disabilities accessing primary health care services. *Journal of Intellectual Disability Research, 50*(1), 11–17.

Mueller, K. J., Ortega, S. T., Parker, K., Patil, K., & Askenazi, A. (1999). Health status and access to care among rural minorities. *Journal of Health Care for the Poor and Underserved, 10*(2), 230–249.

Olkin, R. (1999). The personal, professional and political when clients have disabilities. *Women & Therapy, 22*(2), 87–103.

Piggott, L., Sapey, B., & Wilenius, F. (2005). Out of touch: Local government and disabled people's employment needs. *Disability & Society, 20*(6), 599–611.

Rawlings, E. I., & Carter, D. K. (1977). *Psychotherapy for women: Treatment toward equality.* Springfield, IL: Charles Thomas.

Renzetti, C. M., & Bergen, R. K. (Eds.). (2005). *Violence against women.* Lanham, MD: Rowman & Littlefield.

Root, M. (1996). Women of color and traumatic stress in "domestic capacity": Gender and race as disempowering statuses. In A. J. Marsella, M. J. Friedman, E. T. Gerrity, & R. M. Scurfield (Eds.), *Ethnocultural aspects of posttraumatic stress disorder: Issues, research, and clinical applications* (pp. 363–387). Washington, DC: American Psychological Association.

Sharma, A. (2001). Healing the wounds of domestic abuse: Improving the effectiveness of feminist therapeutic interventions with immigrant and racially visible women who have been abused. *Violence Against Women, 7*(12), 1405–1428.

Smallbone, S. W., & Wortley, R. K. (2004). Onset, persistence, and versatility of offending among adult males convicted of sexual offenses against children. *Sexual Abuse: Journal of Research and Treatment, 16*(4), 285–298.

Weiner, K. M. (1998). Tools for change: Methods of incorporating political/social action into the therapy session. In M. Hill (Ed.), *Feminist therapy as a political act* (pp. 113–123). New York: Haworth Press.

Woolf, S. H., Johnson, R. E., Fryer, G. E., Rust, G., & Satcher, D. (2004). The health impact of resolving racial disparities: An analysis of U.S. mortality data. *American Journal of Public Health, 94*(12), 2078–2081.

CHAPTER 10

Putting It All Together: *Application*

Carolyn West

The metaphor that is used throughout this chapter is chosen from the days of raising my children. During the 1970s, we subscribed to *National Geographic World Magazine* for children, which reliably offered on its back cover magnified close-up photos of some aspect of the natural world. Unnamed, these images were interesting, but confusing, even mysterious. There was always a certain challenge to being able to contextualize these details—to place them in an understandable and meaningful context. It was only from this breadth, from this standing back, from this considered perspective, that the details made sense.

The preceding chapters have made it clear that feminist therapy is an essential and encompassing way of orienting oneself to the practice of therapy. What is also important and what functions to distinguish feminist therapy is that the principles and ethics of feminist therapy as a discipline are necessarily embodied by the feminist therapist as a world orientation. In a shift that may be seen as a radical departure from mainstream therapies, the person of the feminist therapist is not distinct from the practice.

When an individual or family is referred or refers themselves for therapy, there is typically an acknowledgment of the reason, the "why" of referral. Early in mainstream practice, even as a consequence of the initial session, the "how" of therapy, what methods and techniques are to be used, may be established and even required by third parties. But the "who" of therapy related to therapist choice or the person of the therapist is often given minimal attention. As pointed out elsewhere in this volume, a variety of limitations serve to determine which therapist the referred party will see, and to some extent there is an implication that beyond gender preference, a treatment specialty, (e.g., children or trauma), or perhaps, a particular skill set (e.g., EMDR or hypnosis), there is small difference. There is a presumption that if a person has been trained, is properly credentialed, and has the requisite professional experience, therapy can proceed unencumbered, failing only because of the client's resistance or lack of commitment.

But the "who" becomes of critical importance in the domain of feminist therapy because it is the feminist therapist's orientation not simply to the professional field of mental health, but to the sociopolitical and economic structures of the culture and the larger world, that becomes integral to what happens in the therapy office and that overlays and informs the therapist's understanding, interactions, and choices. It is as though the feminist therapist employs a zoom lens that shifts between a wide-angle view of the culture and its forces and a telephoto view that reflects the particular circumstances and histories and strivings of this individual, this couple, this family. And in the movement back and forth between the broad, wide-angle view and the specific, detailed, and personal experience, between situating the client and deconstructing the cultural forces, the feminist therapist works with the client to develop a more finely focused, contextual view of the referral situation—a way of looking and understanding that moves beyond the self and perceived shortcomings to one that is more spacious, and yet more critical, more nuanced, and more empowering.

This concluding application chapter reviews the three cases of Anna and Sergei, Scott and his family, and Abby through a feminist lens, alternately zooming in to consider the particulars of this person and these behaviors and this situation and employing the wide-angle lens to consider them within a sociopolitical and economic context. Although the various factors will be presented in a necessarily linear way, from a feminist framework there are bi-directional connections from the specific to the general and back again among the multiple variables.

ANNA AND SERGEI

With the therapeutic lens focused intently on the presenting issue, it is clear that Anna and Sergei are experiencing multiple stressors, several of which at this point appear to be intense, chronic, and interconnected. Sergei's injury resulted in the loss of health insurance, which not only potentially affects his own health and recovery but also has extremely worrisome consequences in the context of their baby son's life-threatening heart condition and the specialized, ongoing, and high-cost care it necessitates. The realities of a currently limited and unreliable income along with the demands of providing housing, food, and clothing and now medical care also hover over this young family, raising stress levels and portending an uncertain and threatening future.

Additionally, their relatively recent arrival in the United States within an urban neighborhood including few families of Russian origin contributes to a potentially profound sense of isolation. That Anna and Sergei have no extended family in their new country and that they are likewise disconnected from the spiritual and community aspects of their church are conditions further compounding their experience of isolation and vulnerability. An additional element of isolation is suggested by the referral itself in that others in their rental building, rather than offering the support or understanding that might emanate from a neighborly relationship arising out of a sense of shared community, failed to express their concern directly and instead notified social services. At an extraordinary time of layered stress and acute distress, then, Anna and Sergei find themselves alone in a new country, isolated in their immediate living situation, and disconnected from their community and spiritual roots.

With the therapeutic lens focused narrowly, the feminist therapist will also be attentive to what Hill and Jeong in this volume call the "map of the self." Either Anna or Sergei may have innate vulnerabilities to anxiety, for example, or to depression—vulnerabilities that are triggered or exacerbated given the magnitude of their current circumstances. And, as previously pointed out by Ni, their personal histories, individually and as a couple, will shape their experience of and response to what is happening in ways that can be understood by someone else only in the context of a trusting relationship, when there is an invitation to respond to questions that seek out their understanding and experience rather than their perceived failures, and attuned and mindful listening.

Within this listening, too, the feminist therapist will gain an awareness of the strengths of the couple—strengths that can become a foundation for intervention and empowerment. Given what is known about Anna and Sergei, one may conjecture that there is a quality of determination; a willingness to risk; a pride, perhaps, in skilled workmanship; a devotion to family; and the ability to work together as a couple in order to achieve mutual goals.

By broadening the therapeutic lens minimally, a feminist therapist would consider the combination of hesitancy, fear, shame, guilt, and confusion with which this couple may enter therapy. Assuming, in the absence of health insurance and the limited but concrete options offered by most insurers, that social services dictated the arrangements for therapy, the feminist therapist would be conscious of the impact of the overarching as well as the more specific power differentials in this relationship.

It is also unlikely that under these conditions a therapist would be engaged who could join with Anna and Sergei in their own language, thereby leaving them to communicate the emotionally packed and potentially traumatizing details of their experience in a language that may well compromise understanding and increase discomfort. It is further likely that the particular and distancing language of therapy and the intricacies and bureaucracy of social services, rather than bringing relief to the couple, in the short term may actually result in an increase in their distress.

Shifting to a wide-angle lens, the feminist therapist views Anna and Sergei and the circumstances that bring them to therapy against a complex backdrop composed of the myriad of sociocultural and political forces that impact their situation. This practice of contextualization at multiple levels is consistent with the Ballou and Barrett models discussed earlier in this volume. In this case, the major considerations of ethnicity, culture, class, immigrant status, and language intersect to compound the effects of their individual circumstances, compromise their ability to cope effectively or significantly change their situation, and shape in a variety of ways the responses by others at all levels to their plight.

As immigrants, Anna and Sergei are part of a population that has throughout history been marginalized in this country. Their eastern European descent, especially if they lack membership in an ethnic community and the solidarity to which this can give rise, may function to render them largely invisible, a hypothesis that is strongly suggested by the level of their current isolation.

This is also a couple who belong to the working class; who have trades that, without union membership, would afford them only a minimal standard of living; and who may be further marginalized as renters in a culture that reveres ownership as a necessary prerequisite to visibility and status. The failure of the mainstream culture to be able to hear them in their own language seems metaphoric given the realities of their lack of voice in this current circumstance and within the culture in general. It is noteworthy that in spite of a series of highly significant, at best stressful, and potentially traumatic events (e.g., their son's surgeries and Sergei's accident and loss of employment) that would have brought them into contact with and elicited attention from a number of sources, this couple gained visibility only when there was a suspicion of harm to their children—when there was a perception that they may have done something "wrong."

There will also be consideration of ways in which their Russian culture is juxtaposed with the expectations and mode of functioning currently expected of them, much of which is unstated. Their comprehension of how social service agencies work; the role and status of therapy and institutions in their culture; their feelings of powerlessness in the face of hierarchically organized structures; the confusion regarding what to expect or what is expected of them; the likely discomfort, anger, anxiety, and fear evoked by being thrust into a system they do not understand; and the meanings they construct about what is happening based on their own cultural experiences and history are all elements that impact not only how Sergei and Anna will respond but also how they will be responded to.

Each of the exigencies detailed by Hart earlier in this volume concerning matters of referral, the establishment of an alliance with Anna and Sergei, issues of diagnosis and reporting, a way of eliciting the couple's experience that locates the issues within the wide-angle frame, and the identification of goals as a shared task between couple and therapist—each of these will receive attention by a feminist therapist, not because there is a rule book or checklist, but because this is feminist theory made manifest. These are the multiple layers of thinking that define the feminist therapist. As stated by Hill and Jeong, "there is no technique separate from an awareness of political context"—and there is no awareness that is separate from the person of the therapist.

Although the feminist therapist will surely consider a number of possible interventions (see Tabol & Walker, Chapter 6 in this volume), the choices and the manner and degree of investment will emerge cooperatively, resulting in a relationally grounded, shared-power process of "walking with"—a process that contrasts starkly to some more mainstream technique-driven agendas of "doing to." The issue of language flexibility within a context where it is essential to be understood and to understand may arise at the onset of this relationship. Assuming the lack of availability of a therapist who speaks their native language, the feminist therapist may investigate available alternatives, perhaps considering and discussing with the couple any outreach programs established for Russian immigrants from which assistance in translation would be available and viable.

Given the magnitude of the stress this couple is experiencing, the beginning stages of therapy may afford them an opportunity to tell their story and at the same time hear their own story in a way that the immediacy of their situation and the absence of an empathic and attuned ear have previously not invited. Within this telling, a feminist therapist would be supporting Anna and Sergei in examining the broader context of their experience—a process of opening up the lens and situating the particulars of their lives within the framework of their immigrant status, their experience and interface with institutions and agencies, the realities of gaining and retaining employment as immigrants, and the confusion that has likely arisen from conflicting cultural messages about child rearing.

This relationship between feminist therapist and couple, with issues of power named and minimized, would also provide Anna and Sergei a forum for examining their reasons for staying in the United States or returning to Russia, and set within the broader context, what may have been experienced as a sense of personal failure may be freshly understood with the recognition of the impact of significant structural forces on their lives. To the feminist therapist, the political is made personal.

A likely assumption of involved agencies or even a mainstream mental health worker would be that Anna and Sergei should be helped to—and indeed would want to—"assimilate," meaning learn the rules of their station and status and comply with the power structures of the dominant culture. Feminist therapy, on the other hand, by helping to situate their experience within the frame of the dominant culture, would empower Sergei and Anna with clearer vision to make choices that they determine are best for them, including staying in the United States or returning to Russia.

And because facets of their current experience, including the status of their value to the culture beyond their work production, Sergei's lack of employment protection, and loss of critical health care, are directly related to the forces of oppression, the feminist therapist would also seek out groups and programs organized by previous immigrants with whom Anna and Sergei may find solidarity. Not identified in mental health treatment manuals, such solidarity would be an important and powerful "treatment" in this case. Enlarging the frame yet again, the feminist therapist may provide Sergei and Anna with information about the current momentum of immigrant activism in the United States, researching and relaying information about groups and activities accessible to them.

The practice of feminist therapy, then, would move Anna and Sergei from a narrow and constricted place of personal deficit, of failure, of fear and shame, to a more empowered stance from which they can make choices that are in the best interests of themselves and their family. And empowerment for this couple will be accessed through a combination of accurate and relevant information about their new culture, the naming of the sociocultural forces that contribute to their distress, referral to appropriate resources providing both solidarity and support, and a therapist stance that consistently assumes their right to own and chart their life direction.

SCOTT

Feminist therapy in relation to child clients is especially difficult given the obviously limited power of this group. Also, as demonstrated in Scott's case, there are many layers of authority, individuals, and institutions invested in a child's behavior, many or all of which require consideration, including interaction, collaboration, and not infrequently some form of reporting on the part of the therapist. Most frequently, as is true for Scott, children are referred for therapy because of some identified behavior that is thought to be problematic, often a behavior that is viewed as disruptive to some level of group functioning. That children are infrequently if ever in a position to refer themselves and are instead in the position of being "brought to" therapy serves to increase the already enormous power differential between child and therapist and makes the negotiation of the relationship and the boundaries of confidentiality increasingly complex. Yet as described by Pitts, Margolies, and Leeder in Chapter 8, the general approach to feminist therapy with children remains constant, with the intentions to understand the child's experience, support the child's empowerment, and provide advocacy and activism appropriate to the case.

Looking through the lens as it is narrowly focused on the individual, Scott's entry into therapy has been prompted by "a complaint from the school." It seems relevant that this is not framed as a concern for Scott; rather the concern is that Scott is doing something—in this case, covertly tripping other boys in his class and other unspecified ways of "seeking revenge"—that someone, his teacher or other school personnel, wants him to stop. In a generally loving child who seems quite happy at home, these behaviors seem uncharacteristic and suggest some underlying anger or distress that is apparent in the school setting yet directed specifically toward male classmates from whom he has experienced teasing.

Scott's parents frame their concern about Scott quite differently, stating their perception that he has difficulty making friends, particularly males, and describing their efforts to help him become more integrated into a male group while at the same time supporting and affirming his gentle nature.

So in the language of more traditional therapies, what would be considered the "presenting problem" is different depending on who is providing the description. Yet each person or group suggests that there is something about Scott that needs changing—in the first instance, his "aggressive" behavior and in the second instance, his way of expressing gender. As pointed out by Pitts, Margolies, and Leeder, however, Scott himself appears to be doing quite well. His grades are solidly above average, he is engaged with activities of his choice that seem to bring him satisfaction, and he contributes to the running of the household in a willing and age-appropriate manner. Indeed, aside from the parental concern regarding Scott's development in terms of gendered behavior and choices, the family appears to be functioning well.

In widening the lens to place Scott, his school, and his family in the larger social context, however, the undercurrent that precipitates his referral becomes clearer. Although Scott is not demonstrating particular unease with himself, others, from the children in his class to the adults in his family and school, find discomfort in how he presents. Consistent with age and status then, they react either with taunting and marginalization or with complaints about what are really his 9-year-old efforts to defend himself; or with caring concern, they attempt to shape and modify him toward behavior that is more culturally acceptable.

The wide-angle lens used by the feminist therapist reveals Scott against a backdrop of institutionalized gender conformity: the cultural mandate that girls act like girls, that boys behave like boys, and that behavior in a direction of femininity toward "girlie girls" and in a direction of masculinity toward "real boys" is seen and encouraged as "normal" and appropriate. Conversely, behavior in a direction that does not conform to defined gender roles is seen as odd, deviant, or worrisome. It is interesting that the school's complaint about Scott's behavior does not seem to include concern that his male classmates are engaged in acts of harassment; they might see this as just "boys being boys" thereby obviating attention to and intervention for these youngsters.

Individuals—in this case a child—who do not conform to these stereotypes may experience varying degrees of rejection and marginalization, including verbal and physical harassment, victimization, isolation, and potentially traumatic wounding of their sense of self. The institutionalization of gender conformity is engrained throughout the culture, and the penalties for expressing gender in proscribed ways exist on a continuum—from a young boy who may be reprimanded for "crying like a girl" to acts of politically grounded discrimination, socially sanctioned rejection, and acts of violence driven by sexism, non-gender normativity, and heterosexism.

Against this backdrop, the school's reaction to Scott's behavior may be viewed as symptomatic of the larger culture's behavioral proscriptions, and the concern of Scott's family may be seen as a function of their own discomfort with behavior that transverses gender lines, along with their efforts to protect their son from the judgment and consequences of the mainstream culture.

From this culturally situated perspective, a more minor but related issue is Scott's appearance. He is described as tall for his age and about "20 pounds overweight," a status that is likely an additional factor setting him apart from the mainstream notion of masculinity and acceptability. "Chubby" children are teased and bullied, and overweight adults experience widespread rejection and discrimination.

Pitts, Margolies, and Leeder, in Chapter 8 of this volume, provide a considered and comprehensive feminist view of interventions for Scott. Recognizing that the "problem" is situated in the rippling circles of cultural norms that encompass Scott's family, his school and church, his community in the conservative Midwest, and the sociopolitical structures of the mainstream culture and government, rather than in Scott himself, provides the feminist therapist with a framework for their relationship. Rather than colluding with the adults in his world and the culture at large in order to help Scott to fit in, feminist therapy would provide a sensitive, connected listening, an exploration around any action in terms of change that may be seen in collaboration with Scott as consistent with his sense of self, and attention to change—activism—extending into the culture and involving his family, his school, and his community.

It seems important to note that Scott's parents are described as "tolerant of who he is" and as working to provide a secure base in a family that is considered to be "emotionally close." They have made the decision to engage Scott in therapy, a decision that, in a conservative community, may itself be seen as courageous. Additionally, given the father's involvement with the care of the children and his own "gentle" nature, there seems to be an inherent appreciation in this family for some, subtle as it may be, gendered expression that is counter to mainstream norms. Parental support of and participation in Scott's treatment and the potential for their own empowerment and increased ability to advocate for their son are not unrealistic outcomes of the therapeutic relationship.

Yet because children are dependent on an adult to arrange for therapy, to provide transportation, and to maintain the insurance or private payments in order for the therapy to continue and because whether the child gets there or keeps coming rests on some adult's commitment and investment, there is a structural vulnerability built into child work. Additionally, most often, one or more of the adults, as in Scott's case, have a preconceived outcome in mind involving some way in which the child will change as a result of therapy, and not infrequently, this change has to do with how the child will conform better to elements of the mainstream culture. The practice of feminist therapy then must work on multiple fronts to ensure that the child is not withdrawn from therapy prematurely or that the child's increased sense of empowerment and its expression in the environment do not create a greater risk for the individual.

ABBY

Abby arrives in therapy at a time when her anxiety—compelling some recent and demanding checking behaviors—has intruded sufficiently into the functioning of her everyday life such that her normal patterns are obviously and disturbingly disrupted. With the lens focused narrowly and keenly on the individual, it is clear that Abby has been seeking to contain the experience of anxiety at least since her college days, when she discovered that "she liked" the way alcohol with its initially sedative effects made her feel. Her "heavy drinking" may not have stood out as aberrant against the backdrop of college life and in the context of her high grades, but her self-promise to quit after graduation suggests that Abby had a perhaps uneasy awareness of her reliance on this drug.

Without alcohol to temporarily ameliorate her agitation, restlessness, and fear, Abby turned to her primary care physician, who offered her another drug to treat her symptoms. Abby, like many others, relied on this culturally sanctioned, apparently more respectable way of damping down the edges of her anxiety. Managing her symptoms on what appears to be an as-needed but chronic basis, Abby was able to largely avoid or discount the ways in which her beliefs about herself as well as her life choices may have been constricted as a consequence of her early history of abuse.

In Chapter 9 of this volume, Hill and Jeong write, "Many times a person's behavior looks fine to observers, while the individual's internal experience is causing significant suffering." What we know of Abby suggests that she has functioned quite well, even admirably, from an observer's view—attending college, achieving distinctive grades, behaving responsibly regarding her growing reliance on alcohol, and gaining and keeping employment. Yet Abby's internal experience as expressed through the ebb and flow of her anxiety and her attempts to control that which feels unmanageable is one of pain and vulnerability, of shame and isolation.

Although she has long considered and intended that she would be in a relationship and have children, Abby's pattern of isolation and her lack of connectedness, which have developed from and been supported by her internal sense of shame and confusing representations of intimate relationships, function as an invisible yet effective barrier between her and others. Indeed, the consequences of her stepfather's abuse extend well beyond the behaviors that precipitated her Xanax™ prescription or that now bring her to the therapist's office.

Widening the lens to include the sociopolitical frame in which she functions, the feminist therapist views Abby as the foreground in a culturally constructed context, the rules of which are learned implicitly. Against a complex background, it appears that Abby is fulfilling the role that is expected of her as a woman of the middle class. She has successfully separated, or individuated, from her family, she has taken advantage of her socioeconomic class status to attain a college education, and she has become a contributing member of society—that is, she holds a job and supports herself. Consistent with this frame as well, Abby has both minimized and internalized the harm done to her, rather than acknowledging it or naming it as abuse and risking the disapproval of her family. In many ways, Abby fulfills the role of the "good girl": compliant, responsible, conscientious, and unheard.

Although Abby has had access to many of the advantages of the dominant culture, the extent and nature of these advantages and her status within the culture have been diminished by her identity as a person of color. Members of this dominant culture largely consider themselves "color-blind" and dismiss or negate Abby's difficulties in navigating an environment where race continues to affect status and value. She is also female and thus vulnerable to objectification, the injustices of male entitlement, and the range of injuries of oppression and violence experienced by her gender as well as her race. Furthermore, the abuse by her stepfather occurred when Abby was clearly a minor, still dependent physically and emotionally on her parents. As pointed out by Hill and Jeong (this volume), the injustices related to entitlement "may be intertwined with a kind of ownership mentality regarding children." The shame and confusion that would emanate from the abuse by this trusted parental figure has shaped Abby's internal experience of relationships and has been a catalyst for her isolation, her continued self-blame and silence, the arising of her anxious symptomatology, and her vigilant and restricted way of putting herself out into the world.

The following interventions would all be appropriate in a case such as Abby's, but the discussion of what Abby wants to get from the therapy, choices of which interventions and at what point in therapy they would be initiated, will all arise conjointly out of an empathic relationship with her therapist. It is important to note that given the sociopolitical reality of unequal racial access to education, it would be unlikely that Abby would engage with a therapist who herself is a person of color, and so the inherent inequities of the therapeutic relationship would need to be broadened to include this important and definitional factor.

Certainly the immediacy of Abby's escalating and troubling anxiety will be discussed early in the process, along with the possible medical treatment options that can be undertaken in collaboration with her physician. Hart, in this volume, addresses not only the possibility of considering some alternate types of medication but also the critical value in working with Abby to be a self-advocate with her physician in this regard.

Although at least in the short term, Abby will likely benefit from continued psychopharmacological intervention, her therapist may also discuss with her ways in which she can begin to self-manage some of the symptomatology. As with so many victims of sexual abuse, Abby may have become detached from the messages of her body and may be interested in and empowered by learning to recognize the physiological stirrings of anxiety and ways that she can influence the autonomic nervous system on her own behalf. The intersection of relational-cultural therapy and mindfulness meditation may provide access to a new or renewed connection between mind and body for Abby as well as a means for seeing more clearly the relative contributions of forces shaping her anxious reactivity.

But the heart of the intervention for Abby will be in the relationship and in the listening—to this young woman who has not been listened to before and who, indeed, may not have even risked listening nonjudgmentally to herself. As a victim, Abby has likely assumed and internalized the blame for her abuse, and consistent with the sense of shame often experienced by the victims of abuse, she has neither spoken of it nor named it. It is in the therapeutic relationship beyond the management of symptoms that space can be opened for her to express the experience of what happened to her. With the abuse named, the feminist therapist would also situate such abuse within the cultural context of male entitlement—within the wide-angle lens—thereby diminishing shame and the inappropriate assignment of personal responsibility.

Many of the authors in this volume have spoken about the particular feminist principles and the ethics that guide feminist therapy, and in the context of any therapeutic relationship or any intervention, this is assumed. Yet it is important to reiterate that within the therapeutic relationship with Abby, there will be the possibility for her to have a renewed experience of her own value and worthiness and also to experience anew a relationship based in mutual trust and empathy.

The previous chapter also discusses the power inherent in sharing one's experience of trauma and abuse with other women, where group members can listen and speak from a position of personal knowing. Such a format can function as the wide-angle lens, allowing the individual—Abby—to situate her experience within a larger cultural context, reducing self-blame, restoring personal worth, and shattering silence.

Earlier in this volume, within her discussion of the valuing by the feminist therapist of all individuals, Hart presents a thoughtful exploration of the complexity of such relationships as Abby's with her stepfather. The therapist, in the process of supporting Abby and the choices Abby ultimately makes about whether to confront her abuser, also embodies the ways in which human relationships and situations are infused with shadings and texture and not simply this or that—black or white, good or bad—such that Abby need not deny her memories of positive experiences shared with her stepfather in order to own the reality of her abuse and the harm done to her.

For Abby, the empowerment of naming what has happened to her and of confronting her stepfather, if that is what she chooses to do, is in itself a beginning form of activism. She would be placing her abuse in the context of the culture of male entitlement and power over and would be bringing attention to its effects. The feminist therapist would also provide information to Abby about advocacy centers, college programming around issues of abuse, and activist organizations and events, acquaintance with which not only may support her sense of empowerment but also may provide connections and a forum for allowing herself a renewed and fuller place in her world.

The foregoing case analyses apply feminist theory and principles to the work of therapy. This application depends not on a particular skill set, but on the therapist's habitual and honed way of situating the client within multiple, mutually influential contexts. The presenting problem becomes better defined and more clearly understood as it is viewed against the background of socioeconomic and political realities that too often harm and oppress. By employing a continually pulsating lens and moving from the details as captured by the telephoto view to the expanse of the wide-angle picture, the therapist helps the client to understand his or her experience and the breadth of factors influencing the current situation, supports the client in defining and taking action toward his or her goals, and takes an activist stance toward institutions and policies that create and maintain inequity and injustice.

Each of the issues that brought Anna and Sergei, Scott, and Abby, into therapy can be viewed narrowly and neatly as frailties of the individual, and in traditional therapy, they may be treated that way. Feminist therapy situates these same issues within an intricately woven sociocultural fabric even as it considers intervention that regards this as an additional, culturally bound example of injustice.

APPENDIX A

Sample Forms

SAMPLE CLIENT QUESTIONNAIRE

<u>Information Form</u>

Name: _____ Date: _____

Address: _____

_____

Phone (home): _____ Phone (work): _____ Phone (cell): _____

_____

At which numbers is it all right to leave a discreet message? Home: _____ Work: _____

Cell: _____

Date of birth: _____ Social Security Number: _____

Who referred you to me? _____

_____ In case of emergency,

contact: _____ phone: _____

Person responsible for payment (if other than yourself):

Relationship to you: _____

Address: _____

Phone: _____

Please describe the main difficulties that have brought you to see me:

_____

_____

_____

165

Are there stresses in your life that make it more difficult for you to address these problems?

_____

_____

_____

_____

_____

What kinds of things do you do to manage stress, and how are these working in your life now?

_____

_____

_____

_____

_____

Please describe the positive changes you would like to make and what you would like your life to be like:

_____

_____

_____

_____

_____

Have you ever received psychological or psychiatric or counseling services before? Yes_____ No _____

If yes, when? _____

From _____ whom?

For _____ what?

Did you find it helpful? Yes _____ No _____ In what way?

_____

_____

_____

Have you ever taken medications for psychological or emotional problems? Yes ___ No ___
If yes, please indicate:

When?		From whom?		Which medications?		For what reason?		Helpful?	
Yes	No	Yes	No	Yes	No	Yes	No	Yes	No
___	___	___	___	___	___	___	___	___	___
___	___	___	___	___	___	___	___	___	___
___	___	___	___	___	___	___	___	___	___
___	___	___	___	___	___	___	___	___	___

Education
School

Degree	What you studied	When you attended	Graduated?
_____	_____	_____	No ___ Yes ___
_____	_____	_____	No ___ Yes ___
_____	_____	_____	No ___ Yes ___

Have psychological or emotional difficulties ever interfered with school? _____

If yes, please describe: _____

_____

_____

Employment

Employer	Position held/job description	When you worked there
_____	_____	_____
_____	_____	_____
_____	_____	_____
_____	_____	_____

If you are not currently working in paid employment, is this by choice? _____

If no, please explain: _____

_____

Have psychological or emotional difficulties ever interfered with work? _____

_____

If yes, please describe: _____

_____

_____

Relationships and Family
Do you have a significant other/partner? Yes _____ No _____ If yes,
name: _____

Are you married? Yes _____ No _____

How would you describe your sexual orientation?

_____

Please list all those with whom you currently live:

Name	Relationship to you	Are there problems in this relationship?
_____	_____	_____
_____	_____	_____
_____	_____	_____
_____	_____	_____

Do you have children? Yes _____ No _____ If yes, please list their names and ages:

_____

_____

_____

_____

_____

How would you describe your relationship with your children?

_____

_____

_____

_____

_____

Please list the family members with whom you grew up (include family members with whom you may not have lived, but who had an important impact on you [positive or negative] such as a noncustodial parent, a grandparent, etc.):

Name	Relationship to you	Describe the relationship with this person

Have any family members had emotional or psychological problems, or alcohol or drug problems?

Family member's relationship to you	Type of problem

Who are the people in your life *now* with whom you feel closest and/or who provide emotional support?

First name	Relationship to you	How often do you see/talk to this person?	Are there problems in this relationship?

Who have you felt closest to in the past?

First name	Relationship to you	How often did you see/talk to this person?	Were there problems in this relationship?

Are there other sources of emotional support in your life (such as church/religion, a spiritual or intellectual practice, self-help or 12-step program, etc.)?

_____

_____

_____

_____

_____

_____

Do you have a racial or ethnic background that has (or has had in the past) an important impact on your life? Yes ___ No ___ If so, please describe.

_____

_____

_____

_____

_____

_____

_____

Is there anything else you feel it would be helpful for me to know?

_____

_____

_____

_____

_____

_____

_____

_____

This is a strictly confidential record. Redisclosure or transfer is expressly prohibited by law without consent.

CLIENT HEALTH FORM

Health Information

Name: _____   Date: _____

History

1. How would you describe your current health?

   Poor _____ Fair _____ Good _____ Excellent _____

2. Are you having any current health problems?

   Problem   What impact has this problem had on your life?

   _____   _____

   _____   _____

   _____   _____

   _____   _____

   _____   _____

3. Please list any major illnesses, significant accidents and injuries, surgeries, hospitalizations, periods of loss of consciousness, convulsions/seizures, and any other serious medical conditions you have had.

Age	Illness/injury	Treatment received	What was the outcome?
____	_____	_____	_____
____	_____	_____	_____
____	_____	_____	_____
____	_____	_____	_____
____	_____	_____	_____

   What doctors treated you for these?   How do you feel about the care you received?

   _____   _____

   _____   _____

   _____   _____

   _____   _____

   _____   _____

4. What medications (prescribed and over-the-counter) are you taking or have you taken in the last year?

Medication	Dose (how much?)	Condition it is used to treat	Prescribed by
_____	_____	_____	_____
_____	_____	_____	_____
_____	_____	_____	_____
_____	_____	_____	_____

5. Have you done any kinds of work where you were exposed to toxic chemicals?
Yes _____ No _____
If yes, what kinds of chemicals? _____
_____
_____
_____

Medical Caregivers

1. Who is your primary care physician (and who do you see most frequently if different from your PCP)?
_____
_____

Address: _____
_____

Phone number: _____

2. When was your last appointment? _____
_____
_____
_____

3. Have you been happy with the care you receive from your PCP? Yes _____ No _____
If not, why? _____
_____

4. Are you seeing anyone else for health related care, such as a specialist? Yes ____ No ____

Name	Reason for seeing this person	Date of last visit

5. Have you been happy with the care you receive from these specialists? Yes ___ No ___
If not, why? _____
_____

6. Have you had difficulty getting good medical care? Yes ____ No ____ If yes, please explain.
_____
_____
_____
_____

Health Habits

1. What kinds of physical exercise do you get?

_____

_____

_____

_____

2. Do you have any problems getting enough sleep? If yes, please describe the problem.

_____

_____

_____

_____

3. Do you try to restrict your eating in any way or have you in the past? If you have, please say how and why.

_____

_____

_____

_____

Do you have problems with binge eating or purging of any kind, or have you in the past? If yes, please describe.

_____

_____

_____

_____

4. How much coffee, cola, tea, or other sources of caffeine do you consume each day?

_____

_____

_____

_____

5. Do you smoke? If so, how many cigarettes do you smoke each day?

_____

_____

_____

_____

Have you tried to quit and if so how successful were you?

_____

_____

_____

_____

_____

6. How much alcohol do you drink at any one time?

   _____

   What is the most you might drink at one time?

   _____

   How often do you drink?

   _____

   Do you consider your drinking a problem, or have you in the past? If yes, why?

   _____
   _____
   _____
   _____

   Have you ever tried to quit or cut back on your drinking? If yes, were you successful?

   _____
   _____
   _____
   _____

7. Do you use other drugs that are not for a specific medical condition? If so, which ones and how often?

   _____
   _____
   _____
   _____
   _____

   Have you used other drugs in the past? If so, which ones and how often?

   _____
   _____
   _____
   _____

   Do you consider your drug use a problem, either now or in the past? If so, why?

   _____
   _____
   _____
   _____

   Have you ever tried to quit or cut back on your use? If yes, were you successful?

   _____
   _____
   _____
   _____

For Women Only

1. How old were you when you started to menstruate (have your periods)?

_____

_____

How regular are/were your periods?

_____

_____

Has there been much pain with your periods?

_____

_____

Have you noticed mood changes during your cycle?

_____

_____

Have you had any other problems related to your menstrual cycle? If yes, please explain.

_____

_____

2. Have you ever been pregnant?

_____

_____

Have you ever had infertility problems?

_____

_____

Were any of your pregnancies associated with problems other than medical ones (such as being unplanned or the cause of family or relationship problems)?

_____

_____

_____

_____

Your age	Outcome of pregnancy	Any medical problems during the pregnancy or birth (miscarriage, abortion, child born)
_____	_____	_____
_____	_____	_____
_____	_____	_____
_____	_____	_____
_____	_____	_____

If you have had either a miscarriage or an abortion, how did this experience affect you?

_____

_____

_____

3. Have you started menopause? If yes, at what age did the process begin?

_____

_____

_____

What signs or symptoms have you had?

_____

_____

_____

Have you considered these a problem, and if so, in what way?

_____

_____

_____

Other Medical or Physical Problems

Are there any other medical or physical problems with which you are concerned or about which you think it would be helpful for me to know?

_____

_____

_____

Other Health Related Concerns

Is anyone in your family or among your close friends experiencing serious health problems? If yes, please describe these.

_____

_____

_____

Are you providing care for this person in any way?

_____

_____

_____

How is this person's health problem affecting your life (for instance, emotionally, socially, financially)?

_____

_____

_____

This is a strictly confidential record. Redisclosure or transfer is expressly prohibited by law without consent.

INFORMATION ABOUT THERAPY FOR CLIENT UNDERSTANDING/AGREEMENT

SOME INFORMATION ABOUT THERAPY

Therapy is a process of change, usually started by a person who is both in real emotional pain and confused about how to make life better. It always involves two people working together, rather than one doing something to another or telling the other what should be done.

It will be my job as your therapist to help you find the questions you need to ask yourself and to show you new possibilities. I will share my knowledge about psychology and what I have learned from working with others so that you can use this as well as what you know from your own experience to understand yourself and the situation in which you find yourself. Hopefully this will help you make decisions and change the things that are causing you problems.

Therapy can be a very helpful part of making changes in your life. It can help people suffering from depression, anxiety, and other problems with which people struggle, helping them feel more hopeful and less afraid, angry, nervous, or helpless. In therapy, people have a chance to talk things out fully and to experience themselves, the other people in their lives, and the larger world in which they live differently. The process may make their personal goals and values clearer. Therapy can help people recognize the many things that influence their behavior and also help them identify ways to make changes. These changes may help them get more satisfaction out of social and family relationships. They may see ways that they share problems with others in the larger world, letting them feel less isolated and also inspiring them to work toward changes in both their personal social network and the larger world. They may grow in many directions—as individuals, in their close relationships, and in their work or schooling. They may increase their ability to enjoy their lives and reduce their feelings of hopelessness, fear, and powerlessness.

However, therapy can be hard work. People often feel sadness, anxiety, anger, frustration, loneliness, guilt, helplessness, or other uncomfortable feelings while they work on their problems. They may think about painful experiences or memories, and these feelings or thoughts may come up outside of the appointment time. People often enter therapy with problems in their important relationships. Therapy may disrupt these relationships if the person changes in ways that other people do not like. Some people, perhaps including you and some people in your community, may mistakenly view anyone in therapy as weak, or perhaps as seriously disturbed. This is clearly not the case because seeking help and making significant changes require real strength and courage. However, these negative attitudes about people in therapy can affect how easy it is to start and continue therapy.

Because of these things, sometimes a person's problems may seem to temporarily worsen after the beginning of treatment. Most of these difficulties are to be expected when people are making important changes in their lives. However, even with our best efforts, there is a risk that therapy may not help you in the ways you hope it will. I can promise that I will not begin therapy with you if I do not think it will be helpful for you, and I will enter our relationship with optimism about our ability to address your concerns.

During our first sessions we will be doing two things. First, we will work together to find out as much as we can about the problems you are having and about your history and background. It is important that you be as open as you can. However, I also know that many things are very difficult to talk about and that it will take time for some people to feel comfortable with and trust me enough to talk. Please tell me if you are not yet ready to answer a question I ask or to describe painful experiences in depth. In order for us to work together this way, it is important for you to feel comfortable with me, and for us to develop a trusting relationship.

The second thing we will do once we have identified the problem and gotten to know each other a little is develop an initial plan. It is possible that I may recommend that you see someone else if I feel that you need more intensive therapy than I can provide, or if I feel a different therapist would have skills or training that you need and that I do not have. You may also feel that that I am not a good match and ask for a referral. If we both feel comfortable that this is a good fit, we will develop an initial therapy plan.

You have the right to ask any questions you have about your therapy. If you do not understand something I have said or done, or if you disagree with me, *please* tell me. It is important that you understand the process and feel you are making informed decisions. If you want another professional's opinion at any time, or wish to talk with another therapist, I will help you find a qualified person and will provide him or her with the information needed. If you could benefit from a type of therapy I cannot provide, I will help you to get it. You have a right to ask me about other approaches, their risks, and their benefits. Based on what I learn about your problems, I may recommend a medical exam or use of medication. If I do this, I will fully discuss my reasons with you, so that you can decide what is best. If another professional is working with you, I will coordinate my services with her or him and with your own medical doctor, with your permission. Although I do not expect this to happen, if for some reason therapy is not going well, I might suggest you see a different therapist or another professional in addition to, or instead of, me. As a responsible person and ethical therapist, I cannot continue to see you if what we are doing is not working for you.

The length of time you will be in therapy depends on the specific goals you set and on the type of change you are trying to make. Therapy can be short term, lasting a few months, or it can be longer term. I will be able to answer questions about the expected length more easily after we have identified the nature of the problems you are having. Usually sessions are scheduled once per week initially because this allows us to get a better sense of how to work together and make plans about what you will need.

Some Information About Me as Your Therapist

I have been licensed to practice psychology in Pennsylvania since 1986 and have been in private practice since 1990. I received my master's degree from Duquesne University in 1973 and my doctorate from the Pennsylvania State University in 1981. I have a general psychology practice and work with adults of all ages, although I specialize in the issues facing women. I use many approaches in my work, trying to match the approach to each person's individual needs. However, all of my work is tied together by a phenomenological understanding of human experience and by a feminist theoretical perspective on therapy. I am committed to being aware always of the social context in which an individual thinks, feels, and acts and to helping people think of change in broad terms, not just as "fixing" something that is wrong with them individually. If you have any questions about my training or my approach to therapy, please ask.

I have an independent practice, and the nature of the work of a therapist requires that my work be done in private and be unobserved. Although this provides safety and confidentiality for the people in therapy, it also can be problematic for therapists, limiting our ability to recognize our limits or to see new opportunities for change and growth in our work. For this reason I have set up regular consultations with professional colleagues whom I know well and respect for their skill as therapists. I discuss with them my questions and concerns about my work. This helps me keep the quality of my work high, expanding my knowledge and skills and keeping me from being too limited in the way I think about the work I am doing. (Although these colleagues are bound by the same confidentiality requirements as I am, I share only what is necessary to discuss my questions and concerns, and I avoid giving identifying information about individuals. If you would like to know the names of the colleagues with whom I have regular consultations, please ask. I will further restrict what I discuss about your therapy if you ask me to do so.) I am also committed to continuing my understanding of the issues and problems affecting the people with whom I work through continuing education, and I actively pursue this.

What You Can Expect From Our Relationship

As a therapist, I will use my best knowledge and skills to help you. I also have made a commitment to follow the rules and standards of two of the professional organizations to which I belong, the Feminist Therapy Institute and the American Psychological Association. In order to protect the person in therapy, these organizations have developed codes of ethics that outline my obligations as a practicing therapist—for instance, requiring that I continue to learn and improve as a therapist and that I work to improve the world in which I live. These codes also set standards that guide the way therapists interact with those with whom they work. Let me explain some of these, so that you will understand how they affect my interactions with you.

First, it is my responsibility as a therapist to understand the power and influence I can have in the lives of the people with whom I work and to always use this power for their benefit. I am also obligated to recognize and respect the power that each person brings to therapy and to encourage them to recognize and respect their power as well. As a therapist, I must remember that this is not my therapy—it is the other person's—and that I am there to help, not to control or to make decisions for her or him.

Second, I am licensed and trained to practice psychology—not law, medicine, or any other profession. I am not able to give you good advice from these other professional viewpoints.

Third, both state laws and professional ethics codes require me to keep what you tell me confidential (that is, private). You can trust me not to tell anyone else what you tell me, except in certain limited situations. (I will explain more about confidentiality later.)

I also will not reveal in public situations that someone is in therapy with me. This is part of my effort to maintain your privacy. If we meet by chance on the street or in a social situation, I may not say hello or start a conversation with you. This is *not* because I do not want to talk to you, but because

I want to maintain the confidentiality of our relationship. If you say hello to me, I certainly will return your greeting and talk with you. However, I won't discuss things that I know from our therapy sessions in public settings. It is always *your* choice, not mine, whether other people know you are in therapy with me, or even whether others know that I know you.

Fourth, I am obligated to protect and maintain my role as your therapist. According to my professional codes of ethics, I can only be your therapist. I can't be a friend or socialize in private settings with those in therapy with me. I don't accept invitations from clients to social events or family gatherings. I can't be a therapist with someone who is already my friend. I can never have a sexual or romantic relationship with anyone in a therapy relationship with me during, or after, the course of therapy. The ethics codes also place restrictions on most business relationships I can have with people with whom I work, such as using someone as a realtor or hiring someone to work for me. These restrictions on the behavior of the therapist are intended to protect people from any exploitation by therapists (for instance, therapists taking advantage of their influence in the relationship to gain special favors). Most importantly, these restrictions also protect the unique closeness of the therapy relationship. The restriction on friendship relationships between the therapist and the person in therapy is often hard for people to understand, especially because in the course of working together, both often come to like, respect, and care about each other. The restriction is meant to protect the special quality of the therapy relationship: both the therapist and the person in therapy put the needs of that person first and create a safe, private place for this to occur. The person can depend on, open up to, and take risks with the therapist, without worrying about the therapist's personal life and without feeling obligated to the therapist.

Appointments

Therapy sessions are usually 50 minutes long. I will make every effort to be on time, and I ask that you do the same out of consideration for the person whose appointment follows yours. If you must cancel or change an appointment, you need to give me at least 24 hours notice. This will allow me to make your appointment time available to another person. Except for unpredictable emergencies (or situations that both of us would see as an unpredictable emergency), *you will be charged for appointments that are missed without this notice.* (Insurance companies will not reimburse for this fee.)

If phone consultation becomes a regular part of therapy, fees for this will be discussed with you.

Reaching Me by Phone

You can reach me by calling either one of my offices. I have either an answering machine or voice mail for routine messages, and I check these regularly—several times on the day I am in that office and at least once on the day I am not in that office, including weekends. I make every effort to return routine calls within 24 hours of receiving a message, and at least within 48 hours. I have an answering service to take emergency messages. **If you need to reach me in an emergency, or you need to make sure I get your message as soon as possible, please call my answering service at 800-XXX-XXXX.** (The emergency number is also available on the phone messages at both offices.) The staff at the answering service will be able to contact me more directly.

Although I try to be as available as possible, there are times when I cannot be reached immediately, and I do not have a pager. **In case of emergencies when you cannot wait for a return call, please call your local county crisis number (this is listed in the blue pages of the phone book in the Guide to Human Services), or 9-1-1. You can also go to you local emergency room.** If I am out of town, or otherwise unable to return calls, I will have another therapist covering for me. This therapist will be given some information about those with whom I am working in order to make it possible for her to be helpful to someone who calls. She is also bound by the same confidentiality regulations as I am. The staff at the answering service will connect you with this therapist.

Confidentiality

I will treat with great care all the information you share with me. It is your legal right to have my records of our sessions kept private. That is why I ask you to sign an authorization form before I can talk about you or send my records about you to anyone else. Except in the situations discussed in the following paragraphs, I will tell no one what you tell me without your permission. I will not even reveal that you are working with me. (I will be giving you an additional handout about your right to privacy of protected health information.)

Some insurance companies (especially HMOs) require regular updates about treatment for participation in their insurance plan. With an HMO, the insurance company reviews the information I provide in order to determine whether they think therapy is "necessary" and whether to authorize payment for additional sessions. If your insurance company requires this, I will tell you, and we can discuss the information that will be released. These insurance requirements bring up issues of privacy because it can feel to both of us that I am being asked to disclose personal information in order to "prove" that you need therapy. I try to be as sensitive to these issues as possible, and I will work with you so that you can protect your privacy from unnecessary intrusions.

Almost all insurance companies require that I give them a diagnosis and that you sign an authorization to the release of information in order to receive reimbursement. Starting April 14, 2003, new federal regulations for the privacy and security of protected health information (HIPAA) distinguish between your clinical record (which both you and others such as an insurance company may have the right to access as a condition of payment) and psychotherapy notes (which are for my use only). The clinical record includes diagnosis, therapy plan, prognosis, progress notes, medication information, and social and medical history, but does not need to include details of what we discuss in our sessions. I am required by law to keep a record including this information for each session I have with you.

You have a right to see any information in your medical record. I do not routinely keep separate psychotherapy notes, but I may do this for some people. These types of notes are intended for my use only and consist of my thoughts and reflections about the session or the process of therapy and details that I want to remember. Under the new federal laws, psychotherapy notes are not available to anyone else besides me (including the person with whom I am working) and are kept separate from the medical record. However, it is not clear whether they might be subject to disclosure if a court order is issued because the new law has not been challenged in court. For this reason I am careful about what I include in notes and do not record more detail than is necessary for good therapy.

Some insurance plans also require that I communicate with your primary care physician unless there is a documented reason for not doing so. This is often helpful, especially if your doctor referred you to me, if there are medical conditions that may be related to your problems or your therapy, or if you are taking medication. However, it is ultimately your decision whether I share information with anyone, and the insurance company will not refuse payment if you object.

In all but a few rare situations, your confidentiality is protected by state law, by federal privacy regulations, and by the rules of my profession. Here are the most common cases in which confidentiality is *not* protected:

1. If you make a serious threat to harm yourself or another person, the law requires me to try to protect you or that other person. This may mean telling others about the threat. I cannot promise never to tell someone if I think you are going to hurt yourself or somebody else.
2. If I believe a child has been or will be abused or neglected, I am ethically required to report this.

3. If I have reason to believe that an elderly person or other adult is in need of protective services (because of abuse, neglect, exploitation, or abandonment), the law allows me to report this to appropriate authorities, usually the Department of Aging in the case of an elderly person. Once such a report is filed, I may be required to provide additional information.

4. If you were sent to me by a court for evaluation or therapy, I am actually working for the court and will have to provide reports to the court, probation office, or other agency. If this is your situation, please talk with me before you tell me anything you do not want the court to know. You have a right to tell me only what you feel safe telling me. However, this often complicates or prevents effective therapy.

5. If you are involved in a court proceeding, and a request is made for information concerning the professional services I provided to you, such information is protected by privilege laws and normally requires your written authorization. However, I can be compelled to produce records by a court order under some circumstances. If you are involved in or contemplating litigation, you should consult with your attorney to determine whether a court would be likely to order me to disclose information.

6. If a government agency (such as Medicare) is requesting the information for health oversight activities, I may be required to provide it.

7. If I am seeing someone who files a worker's compensation claim, I may, upon appropriate request, be required to provide otherwise confidential information to the person's employer.

If one of these situations arises, I will make every effort to discuss it with you before taking any action and to limit my disclosure to what is necessary for the situation.

There are two situations in which I might talk about part of our work together with another therapist. First, when I am away from the office for a few days, I will ask another trusted therapist to "cover" for me. This therapist will be available to you in emergencies. Therefore, she may need to know about you. Generally, I will tell this therapist only what she or he would need to know for an emergency. Of course, this therapist is bound by the same laws and rules as I am to protect your confidentiality.

Second, when I consult other therapists or other professionals about the work I do, some information is shared. These professionals are bound by the same confidentiality requirements as I am and are also required to keep your information private. Your name will not be given to them without your specific permission, and they will be told only as much as they need to know to understand your situation and the work we are doing.

Except for the situations I have just described, I will always maintain your privacy, and any office staff that has to work with your information is bound by the same requirement. Everyone who has contact with your records (for instance, doing filing) signs a formal contract in which they promise to maintain confidentiality.

Although you are not bound by the same legal requirements, I also ask you not to disclose the name or identity of anyone you happen to see in my office.

Fees and Payments

Fees will be discussed with you either before or during your first appointment and will be listed on the consent to treatment that I will ask you to sign. Payment is expected at the time of your appointment unless specific arrangements have been made. I will provide monthly statements for you that can be submitted to your insurance company for reimbursement or kept for tax records. It will show all of our meetings, the charges for each, how much has been paid, and how much (if anything) is still owed.

Most insurance companies cover my services, but I cannot guarantee payment by any insurance company because plans vary widely. Please check with your company about coverage. If I am a contracted therapist with an insurance company, I may be required to accept less than my usual fee as a condition of participation in the company's network. I will make it clear what your co-pay is in these situations.

If you need help with your insurance forms, please ask. Some companies require that I bill them directly; we will discuss this either before or at our first meeting.

If I increase my fee during the time we are working together, I will discuss this with you before the change is effective. However, your co-payment or deductible may be determined by your particular health plan and may change without my knowledge.

If problems arise with payment because of changes in your circumstances, please talk to me as soon as possible. Please do not cancel appointments or end therapy for financial reasons without talking to me first.

Reduced Fees

I reserve a certain number of appointment times each week for those who cannot afford to pay the full fee for psychotherapy. I strongly believe that the opportunity to receive help for psychological problems should not be as dependent on income or on the availability of adequate health insurance as it is in our country.

I also believe that we are all dependent on one another because we live in a community—in supporting others, we are also supporting ourselves. Providing my services at a reduced fee is one way of meeting my responsibility to my community and of acknowledging the support I have received and continue to receive from others. However, I also recognize that accepting a reduced fee may bring up other problems for some people, given that accepting this kind of support is often seen as weak or shameful in our society. Those who know they are paying less for their therapy than others may feel like they 'owe" me something and may also feel less free to question or disagree with me. In this less-than-ideal world, it is often difficult to feel like someone is our equal if we do not have the same financial status, if we think we owe someone, or if we feel dependent. This can make it difficult for us to work as full partners in therapy. Although we may not be able to eliminate these feelings and attitudes completely, we can work together to reduce the way they interfere with therapy.

Court Testimony

If you ever become involved in a divorce or custody dispute or other legal dispute, I want you to understand that I do not provide evaluations or expert testimony in court. You should hire a different mental health professional for any evaluations or expert testimony you require. This position is based on several reasons: (1) I am not trained in family or custody evaluations or as a forensic psychologist; (2) my statements will most likely be seen as biased because we have a therapy relationship; and (3) the testimony might negatively affect our therapy relationship, and I want to put this relationship first.

Statement of Principles and Complaint Procedures

In my practice as a therapist, I do not discriminate against clients because of any of these factors: age, sex, race, color, sexual orientation, gender identification, religious beliefs, ethnic origin, social class or income status, place of residence, physical disability, health status, marital/family status, veteran status, or criminal record unrelated to present dangerousness.

This is a personal commitment, as well as being required in part by federal, state, and local laws and regulations. I will always take steps to advance and support the values of equal opportunity, human dignity, and diversity in our community. If you believe that I have acted in a way that is not consistent with this commitment (that I have discriminated against you in any way or devalued or ignored your experience), *please* bring this matter to my attention imme-diately. It is inevitable that you and I will have experiences and backgrounds that differ in some important ways, and I will make a real effort to understand and be sensitive to these differences. If you feel I have not succeeded in *any* way, please tell me.

I fully abide by all the ethics codes of the Feminist Therapy Institute (available at its website: www.feministtherapyinstitute.org) and the American Psychological Association (APA) and by those of my state license. (The APA's rules include its Ethical Principles, its Standards for Providers of Psychological Services, and its Guidelines for Delivery of Specialty Services by Clinical Psychologists.)

Problems can arise in our relationship, just as in any other relationship. If you are not satisfied with any area of our work, please raise your concerns with me at once. Our work together will be slower and harder if these issues are not worked out. I will make every effort to hear any complaints you have and to seek solutions to them. If you feel that I, or any other therapist, have treated you unfairly or have broken a professional rule, please tell me. You can also contact the state or local psychological association (the Pennsylvania Psychological Association, 717-232-3817, and the Central Pennsylvania Psychological Association) and speak to the chairperson of the ethics committee. He or she can help clarify your concerns or tell you how to file a complaint. You may also contact the State Board of Psychology, the organization that licenses those of us in the independent practice of psychology.

Again, *please* make sure you ask me any questions you have about what I have written here, or about anything in your therapy. Also, I really want you to make any suggestions you have (now or later) about how we can work together effectively. I truly appreciate the chance you have given me to work with you, and I look forward to our therapy together.

APPENDIX B

Feminist Therapy Institute
Code of Ethics* (Revised, 1999)

PREAMBLE

Feminist therapy evolved from feminist philosophy, psychological theory and practice, and political theory. In particular feminists recognize the impact of society in creating and maintaining the problems and issues brought into therapy.

Briefly, feminists believe the personal is political. Basic tenets of feminism include a belief in the equal worth of all human beings, a recognition that each individual's personal experiences and situations are reflective of and an influence on society's institutionalized attitudes and values, and a commitment to political and social change that equalizes power among people. Feminists are committed to recognizing and reducing the pervasive influences and insidious effects of oppressive societal attitudes and society.

Thus, a feminist analysis addresses the understanding of power and its interconnections among gender, race, culture, class, physical ability, sexual orientation, age, and anti-Semitism as well as all forms of oppression based on religion, ethnicity, and heritage. Feminist therapists also live in and are subject to those same influences and effects and consistently monitor their beliefs and behaviors as a result of those influences.

Feminist therapists adhere to and integrate feminist analyses in all spheres of their work as therapists, educators, consultants, administrators, writers, editors, and/or researchers. Feminist therapists are accountable for the management of the power differential within these roles and accept responsibility for that power. Because of the limitations of a purely intrapsychic model of human functioning, feminist therapists facilitate the understanding of the interactive effects of the client's internal and external worlds. Feminist therapists possess knowledge about the psychology of women and girls and utilize feminist scholarship to revise theories and practices, incorporating new knowledge as it is generated.

Feminist therapists are trained in a variety of disciplines, theoretical orientations, and degrees of structure. They come from different cultural, economic, ethnic, and racial backgrounds. They work in many types of settings with a diversity of clients and practice different modalities of therapy, training, and research. Feminist therapy theory integrates feminist principles into other theories of human development and change.

The ethical guidelines that follow are additive to, rather than a replacement for, the ethical principles of the profession in which a feminist therapist practices. Amid this diversity, feminist therapists are joined together by their feminist analyses and perspectives. Additionally, they work toward incorporating feminist principles into existing professional standards when appropriate.

Feminist therapists live with and practice in competing forces and complex controlling interests. When mental health care involves third-party payers, it is feminist therapists' responsibility to advocate for the best possible therapeutic process for the client, including short or long term therapy. Care and compassion for clients include protection of confidentiality and awareness of the impacts of economic and political considerations, including the increasing disparity between the quality of therapeutic care available for those with or without third-party payers.

Feminist therapists assume a proactive stance toward the eradication of oppression in their lives and work toward empowering women and girls. They are respectful of individual differences, examining oppressive aspects of both their own and clients' value systems. Feminist therapists engage in social change activities, broadly defined, outside of and apart from their work in their professions. Such activities may vary in scope and content but are an essential aspect of a feminist perspective.

This code is a series of positive statements that provide guidelines for feminist therapy practice, training, and research. Feminist therapists who are members of other professional organizations adhere to the ethical codes of those organizations. Feminist therapists who are not members of such organizations are guided by the ethical standards of the organization closest to their mode of practice.

These statements provide more specific guidelines within the context of and as an extension of most ethical codes. When ethical guidelines are in conflict, the feminist therapist is accountable for how she prioritizes her choices.

These ethical guidelines, then, are focused on the issues feminist therapists, educators, and researchers have found especially important in their professional settings. As with any code of therapy ethics, the well-being of clients is the guiding principle underlying this code. The feminist therapy issues that relate directly to the client's well-being include cultural diversities and oppressions, power differentials, overlapping relationships, therapist accountability, and social change. Even though the principles are stated separately, each interfaces with the others to form an interdependent whole. In addition, the code is a living document and thus is continually in the process of change.

The Feminist Therapy Institute's Code of Ethics is shaped by economic and cultural forces in North America and by the experiences of its members. Members encourage an ongoing international dialogue about feminist and ethical issues. It recognizes that ethical codes are aspirational and ethical behaviors are on a continuum rather than reflecting dichotomies. Additionally, ethical guidelines and legal requirements may differ. The Feminist Therapy Institute provides educational interventions for its members rather than disciplinary activity.

The Feminist Therapy Institute, Inc.
Administrator: Marcia Chappell
912 Five Islands Rd
Georgetown, ME 04548
INFO@FEMINISTTHERAPYINSTITUTE.ORG

Ethical Guidelines for Feminist Therapists

I. CULTURAL DIVERSITIES AND OPPRESSIONS

A. A feminist therapist increases her accessibility to and for a wide range of clients from her own and other identified groups through flexible delivery of services. When appropriate, the feminist therapist assists clients in accessing other services and intervenes when a client's rights are violated.

B. A feminist therapist is aware of the meaning and impact of her own ethnic and cultural background, gender, class, age, and sexual orientation, and actively attempts to become knowledgeable about alternatives from sources other than her clients. She is actively engaged in broadening her knowledge of ethnic and cultural experiences, nondominant and dominant.

C. Recognizing that the dominant culture determines the norm, the therapist's goal is to uncover and respect cultural and experiential differences, including those based on long term or recent immigration and/or refugee status.

D. A feminist therapist evaluates her ongoing interactions with her clientele for any evidence of her biases or discriminatory attitudes and practices. She also monitors her other interactions, including service delivery, teaching, writing, and all professional activities. The feminist therapist accepts responsibility for taking action to confront and change any interfering, oppressing, or devaluing biases she has.

II. POWER DIFFERENTIALS

A. A feminist therapist acknowledges the inherent power differentials between client and therapist and models effective use of personal, structural, or institutional power. In using the power differential to the benefit of the client, she does not take control or power which rightfully belongs to her client.

B. A feminist therapist discloses information to the client which facilitates the therapeutic process, including information communicated to others. The therapist is responsible for using self-disclosure only with purpose and discretion and in the interest of the client.

C. A feminist therapist negotiates and renegotiates formal and/or informal contacts with clients in an ongoing mutual process. As part of the decision-making process, she makes explicit the therapeutic issues involved.

D. A feminist therapist educates her clients regarding power relationships. She informs clients of their rights as consumers of therapy, including procedures for resolving differences and filing grievances. She clarifies power in its various forms as it exists within other areas of her life, including professional roles, social/governmental structures, and interpersonal relationships. She assists her clients in finding ways to protect themselves and, if requested, to seek redress.

III. OVERLAPPING RELATIONSHIPS

A. A feminist therapist recognizes the complexity and conflicting priorities inherent in multiple or overlapping relationships. The therapist accepts responsibility for monitoring such relationships to prevent potential abuse of or harm to the client.

B. A feminist therapist is actively involved in her community. As a result, she is aware of the need for confidentiality in all settings. Recognizing that her client's concerns and general well-being are primary, she self-monitors both public and private statements and comments. Situations may develop through community involvement where power dynamics shift, including a client having equal or more authority than the therapist. In all such situations a feminist therapist maintains accountability.

C. When accepting third party payments, a feminist therapist is especially cognizant of and clearly communicates to her client the multiple obligations, roles, and responsibilities of the therapist. When working in institutional settings, she clarifies to all involved parties where her allegiances lie. She also monitors multiple and conflicting expectations between clients and care-givers, especially when working with children and elders.

D. A feminist therapist does not engage in sexual intimacies nor any overtly or covertly sexualized behaviors with a client or former client.

IV. THERAPIST ACCOUNTABILITY

A. A feminist therapist is accountable to herself, to colleagues, and especially to her clients.

B. A feminist therapist will contract to work with clients and issues within the realm of her competencies. If problems beyond her competencies surface, the feminist therapist utilizes consultation and available resources. She respects the integrity of the relationship by stating the limits of her training and providing the client with the possibilities of continuing with her or changing therapists.

C. A feminist therapist recognizes her personal and professional needs and utilizes ongoing self-evaluation, peer support, consultation, supervision, continuing education, and/or personal therapy. She evaluates, maintains, and seeks to improve her competencies, as well as her emotional, physical, mental, and spiritual well being. When the feminist therapist has experienced a similar stressful or damaging event as her client, she seeks consultation.

D. A feminist therapist continually re-evaluates her training, theoretical background, and research to include developments in feminist knowledge. She integrates feminism into psychological theory, receives ongoing therapy training, and acknowledges the limits of her competencies.

E. A feminist therapist engages in self-care activities in an ongoing manner outside the work setting. She recognizes her own needs and vulnerabilities as well as the unique stresses inherent in this work. She demonstrates an ability to establish boundaries with the client that are healthy for both of them. She also is willing to self-nurture in appropriate and self-empowering ways.

V. SOCIAL CHANGE

A. A feminist therapist seeks multiple avenues for impacting change, including public education and advocacy within professional organizations, lobbying for legislative actions, and other appropriate activities.

B. A feminist therapist actively questions practices in her community that appear harmful to clients or therapists. She assists clients in intervening on their own behalf. As appropriate, the feminist therapist herself intervenes, especially when other practitioners appear to be engaging in harmful, unethical, or illegal behaviors.

C. When appropriate, a feminist therapist encourages a client's recognition of criminal behaviors and also facilitates the client's navigation of the criminal justice system.

D. A feminist therapist, teacher, or researcher is alert to the control of information dissemination and questions pressures to conform to and use dominant mainstream standards. As technological methods of communication change and increase, the feminist therapist recognizes the socioeconomic aspects of these developments and communicates according to clients' access to technology.

E. A feminist therapist, teacher, or researcher recognizes the political is personal in a in a world where social change is a constant.

Index

SPRINGER PUBLISHING COMPANY

Abortion Counseling

A Clinician's Guide to Psychology, Legislation, Politics, and Competency

Rachel B. Needle, PsyD
Lenore E. A. Walker, EdD

Foreword by Nancy Felipe Russo, PhD

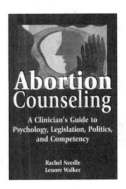

"Abortion counseling has a critical role to play in ensuring women's mental health is the priority and not the goal of a political agenda. Thus, Needle and Walker have taken on a complex, profound, and essential task— equipping therapists and abortion counselors with the knowledge and skills needed to help their clients—and they have done it well....

"Readers of this book should [gain] an increased understanding of how women's diverse life circumstances affect their ability to cope with the difficult decisions and circumstances surrounding abortion. They will also be better able to build women's resilience and coping skills by having considered them both in the context of women's lives (e.g., coping resources, social support, partner violence, incidence of depression), and in the context of sociopolitical agendas that seek to manipulate women's mental health in order to undermine women's reproductive rights....In the final analysis, it is important to remember that abortion counseling is not about abortion—it is about women confronting the decision to bear a child—with all of the profound and life-changing commitments and responsibilities that entails."

—From the Foreword by **Nancy Felipe Russo,** PhD,
Regents Professor of Psychology, Arizona State University

Through this book the authors hope to train general therapists and counselors in pre- and post-abortion counseling techniques—to avoid women experiencing unnecessary psychological problems created by those who insist that the nonexistent "post-abortion syndrome" exists.

2007 · 288pp · softcover · 978-0-8261-0257-7

11 West 42nd Street, New York, NY 10036-8002 • Fax: 212-941-7842
Order Toll-Free: 877-687-7476 • Order Online: www.springerpub.com

SPRINGER PUBLISHING COMPANY

Depression and Women
An Integrative Treatment Approach
Susan L. Simonds, PhD

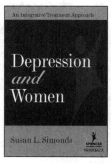

"This book carries on the fine feminist tradition of looking at women's unique treatment needs in a manner that will illuminate, in important ways, the treatment of women's depression. Simonds does a masterful job of presenting a feminist perspective on the empowerment of depressed women, who experience themselves as powerless, and does so in a highly accessible manner that will make this volume useful to therapists from many theoretical perspectives. If you work with depressed women, this will be necessary reading from now on."

—**Laura S. Brown**, PhD, ABPP
Director, Fremont Community Therapy Project
Seattle, WA

The book provides comprehensive reviews of the literature including the epidemiology and causes of women's depression, treatment of depression outcome studies, special medication issues for women, and reproductive-related depression. The author provides a practical, user-friendly approach to the treatment of depressed women and includes chapters on the client who is not improving, relapse prevention, and therapist self-care. A valuable resource for therapists, psychologists, clinical social workers, and graduate students in psychology.

Partial Contents:

- Integrative Relational Therapy With Depressed Women: Basic Assumptions
- Why Are So Many Women Depressed?
- What Can We Learn From Treatment Outcome Studies?

- The Therapeutic Relationship and Special Issues With Women
- Assessment: Philosophy and Standards of Care
- Assessment: Case Conceptualization
- Safety
- Activation

- Connection: Part I
- Connection: Part II
- Meaning
- Relapse Prevention
- When the Client Is Not Improving
- Therapist Self-Care
- Appendix A
- References

2006 · 304pp · softcover · 978-0-8261-1444-0

11 West 42nd Street, New York, NY 10036-8002 • Fax: 212-941-7842
Order Toll-Free: 877-687-7476 • Order Online: www.springerpub.com